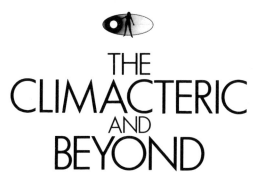

THE
CLIMACTERIC
AND
BEYOND

THE
CLIMACTERIC
AND
BEYOND

The Proceedings of the Fifth International Congress on the
Menopause, held in Sorrento (Italy), 6–10 April, 1987, under
the auspices of the International Menopause Society

The Proceedings include the Keynote Address, Plenary
Lectures and the Workshop
Reports presented during this Congress

Edited by
L. Zichella, M. I. Whitehead and P. A. van Keep

The Parthenon Publishing Group
International Publishers in Science & Technology

Casterton Hall, Carnforth,
Lancs, LA6 2LA, U.K.

120 Mill Road, Park Ridge
New Jersey, U.S.A.

Published in the U.K. and Europe by
The Parthenon Publishing Group Ltd.
Casterton Hall
Carnforth, Lancs. LA6 2LA   — ISBN 1 85070 176 8

Published in the USA by
The Parthenon Publishing Group Inc.
120 Mill Road
Park Ridge, New Jersey 07656 USA   — ISBN 0 940813 06 8

Printed in Great Britain by
Butler & Tanner Ltd, Frome and London

Contents

Section 2 Workshop Reports

List of principal contributors

DR S. BALLINGER

University of Sydney, Dept. Behavioural Sciences in Medicine, Sydney, NSW 2006, Australia.

PROF S. BELISLE

University of Sherbrooke, Dept. Obstet. and Gynaecology, Faculty of Medicine, Central Hospital, Sherbrooke, Quebec J1H 5N4, Canada.

DR E. BORSTAD

Dept. Obstetrics and Gynaecology, Aker Sykehus, 0514 Oslo 5, Norway.

A. BRANDBERG, M.D.

Sahlgrenska Sjukhuset, Mikrobiologiska Laboratorierna, Guldhedsgatan 10, 413 46 Goeteborg, Sweden.

PROF C. CHRISTIANSEN

University of Copenhagen, Glostrup Hospital, Dept. Clinical Chemistry, Nordre Ringvej, 2600 Glostrup, Denmark.

D. W. CRAMER, M.D.

Harvard Medical School, Dept. Obstetrics-Gynecology, Brigham and Women's Hospital, 75 Francis Street, Boston, MA 02115, U.S.A.

DR N. CRONA

Sahlgrenska Hospital, Kvinnokliniken, 413 45 Goeteborg, Sweden.

DR M. CUST

Academic Department of Obstetrics and Gynaecology, King's College School of Medicine and Dentistry, Denmark Hill, London SE5 8RX, United Kingdom.

L. FÅHRAEUS, M.D.

University Hospital, Dept. Obstetrics and Gynaecology, 581 85 Linkoeping, Sweden.

DR D. FRASER

Menopause Clinic, King's College School of Medicine and Dentistry, Denmark Hill, London SE5 8RX, United Kingdom.

PROF H. K. GENANT

University of California, Dept. Radiology, Medicine and Orthopaedic Surg., M-396, San Francisco, CA 94143, U.S.A.

PROF A. R. GENAZZANI

Università degli Studi di Modena, Istituto di Clinica Ostetrica e Ginecologica, Policlinico, Via del Pozzo 71, 41100 Modena, Italy.

PROF C. GENNARI

Università di Siena, Istituto di Semeiotica Medica, Piazza Duomo 2, 53100 Siena, Italy.

J. GINSBURG, M.D.

Consultant Endocrinologist, Royal Free Hospital Medical School, Pond Street, London NW3 2QG, United Kingdom.

DR L. GOOREN

VU Academisch Ziekenhuis, Div. Andrology/Endocrinology, Dept. Internal Medicine, P.O. Box 7057, 1007 MB Amsterdam, Netherlands.

PROF R. B. GREENBLATT

Medical College of Georgia, School of Medicine, Dept. Physiology and Endocrin., 903 15th Street, Augusta, Georgia 30910-0192, U.S.A.

DR J. G. GREENE

Gartnavel Royal Hospital, Dept. Clinical Psychology, 1055 Great Western Road, Glasgow G12 0XH, United Kingdom.

G. HEIMER, M.D.

University Hospital, Dept. Obstetrics and Gynaecology, 750 14 Uppsala 14, Sweden.

PROF E. HIRVONEN

University Central Hospital, Dept. I and II Obstetrics and Gynaecology, Bulevardi 22 A, 00120 Helsinki, Finland.

PROF A. HOLTE

University of Oslo, Institute of Behavioural Sciences in Medicine, P.O. Box 1111, Blindern, 0317 Oslo 3, Norway.

DR M. HUNTER

King's College Hospital, Dept. Psychological Medicine, Denmark Hill, London SE5 9RS, United Kingdom.

P. A. VAN KEEP, M.D.

International Menopause Society, 8 Avenue Don Bosco, 1150 Brussels, Belgium.

PROF R. LINDSAY

Helen Hayes Hospital, Bone Metabolism Unit, Route 9W, West Haverstraw, New York, NY 10993, U.S.A.

R. A. LOBO, M.D.

University of Southern California, School of Medicine, Dept. Obstetrics-Gynecology, Women's Hospital, Room 1M2, 1240 North Mission Road, Los Angeles, California 90033, U.S.A.

DR M. LOCK

McGill University, Dept. Humanities and Social Studies, 3655 Drummond Street, Montreal, PQ H3G 1Y6, Canada.

PROF L. E. MARKS

John B. Pierce Foundation Laboratory, 290 Congress Avenue, New Haven, Connecticut 06519, U.S.A.

PROF G. F. MAZZUOLI

4. Patologia Medica, c/o 2. Clinica Medica Policlinico Umberto 1, Università la Sapienza, 00161 Rome, Italy.

DR G. B. MELIS

Università di Pisa, Clinica Ostetrica e Ginecologica, Osp. Riuniti S. Chiara, Via Roma 67, 56100 Pisa, Italy.

PROF L. J. MELTON, III

Mayo Clinic, Dept. Medical Statistics and Epidemiology, 200 First Street SW, Rochester, Minnesota 55905, U.S.A.

F. PETRAGLIA, M.D.

Università Degli Studi di Modena, Istituto Clinica Ostetrica e Ginecologica, Via del Pozzo 71, 41100 Modena, Italy.

H. REKERS, M.D.

International Health Foundation, 8 Avenue Don Bosco, 1150 Brussels, Belgium.

PROF J. RESNICK

University of Florida, Psychology and Vocational Counselling Center, 311 Little Hall, Gainesville, Florida 32611, U.S.A.

R. K. ROSS, M.D.

University of Southern California, School of Medicine, Dept. Preventive Medicine, 2025 Zonal Ave., Noris 803, Los Angeles, California 90033, U.S.A.

DR R. RUBENS

Rijksuniversiteit Gent, Afd. Endocrinologie-Haematologie-Stofwisselingsziekten, De Pintelaan 185, 9000 Ghent, Belgium.

T. RUD, M.D.

Dept. Obstetrics and Gynaecology, Aker Sykehus, 0514 Oslo 5, Norway.

P. M. SARREL, M.D.

Yale University Health Services, Dept. Obstetrics-Gynecology-Psychiatry, 17 Hillhouse Avenue, New Haven, Connecticut 06520, U.S.A.

B. VON SCHOULTZ, M.D.

University of Umea, Dept. Obstetrics and Gynaecology, 901 85 Umea, Sweden.

DR S. SCHWARTZ-GIBLIN

The Rockefeller University, Laboratory of Neurobiology and Behavior, 1230 York Avenue, New York, NY 10021-6399, U.S.A.

R. SITRUK-WARE, M.D.

Ciba Geigy Ltd, Central Medical Affairs, K490, 3, 37, 4002 Basle, Switzerland.

DR J. C. STEVENSON

H.D.D.R., Cavendish Clinic, 21 Wellington Road, London NW8 9SQ, United Kingdom.

MR J. STUDD

Dulwich Hospital, Menopause Clinic. Mailing Address: 120 Harley Street, London W1N 1AG, United Kingdom.

A.-Z. TERAN, M.D.

Medical College of Georgia, Dept. Endocrinology, Augusta, Georgia 30912, U.S.A.

R. TUIMALA, M.D.

University Central Hospital, Dept. Gynaecology, 33520 Tampere 52, Finland.

G. V. UPTON, Ph.D.

Wyeth Laboratories, Clinical Research and Development, P.O. Box 8299, Philadelphia, PA 19101-8299, U.S.A.

W. H. UTIAN, M.D.

Mt. Sinai Medical Center, Dept. Obstetrics and Gynecology, University Circle, Cleveland, OH 44106, U.S.A.

PROF M. VESSEY

Oxford University, Dept. Community Medicine and General Practice, Radcliffe Infirmary, Oxford OX2 6HE, United Kingdom.

A. VICTOR, M.D.

Uppsala University, Dept. Obstetrics and Gynaecology, 751 85 Uppsala, Sweden.

M. I. WHITEHEAD, M.D.

King's College School of Medicine and Dentistry, Dept. Obstetrics-Gynaecology, Denmark Hill, London SE5 8RX, United Kingdom.

PROF D. DE WIED

Rudolf Magnus Institute for Pharmacology, Medical Faculty of the University of Utrecht, Vondellaan 6, 3521 GD Utrecht, Netherlands.

DR TJ. B. VAN WIMERSMA GREIDANUS

Rudolf Magnus Institute for Pharmacology, Medical Faculty of the University of Utrecht, Vondellaan 6, 3521 GD Utrecht, Netherlands.

B. G. WREN, M.D.

Centre Management Menopause, Under Auspices Benevolent Society NSW, Royal Hospital for Women, Renwick House, 1st floor, Paddington, NSW 2021, Australia.

PROF L. ZICHELLA

I Clinica Ostetrica e Ginecologica, "La Sapienza", Policlinico Umberto I, 00161 Rome, Italy.

Preface

Interest in the female menopause and its sequelae is growing steadily. This is reflected in the increasing numbers of participants that the three-yearly congresses of the International Menopause Society attract.

The Fifth International Congress on the Menopause was held in Sorrento (Italy) from 6 to 10 April 1987. This volume contains the Keynote Address, most of the papers presented at the Plenary Sessions and the reports of all the Workshop chairpersons. The Editors regret that they were unable to make this book entirely complete, but any further delay in publication would have diminished the value of the information presented here.

The lectures delivered at the Plenary Sessions are shown in the order they were presented during the Congress and so are the Workshop reports.

One of the papers is by Robert Greenblatt, Honorary President of the International Menopause Society, who passed away at the time that these proceedings went into print. The Editors, who were also involved in drafting the Congress Programme, wish to record their gratitude for the valuable contribution he made both to the Congress and to this publication.

The International Menopause Society set out as a Society whose aim was to further the study of the climacteric in both sexes. Consequently, one workshop was devoted to the male climacteric and time was reserved for special communications on this subject. However, only very few abstracts on this topic were submitted. Clearly, it is the female menopause which constitutes the centre of interest of the members of the Society.

The Editors' thanks are due not only to Mrs Fredy Makkes, who handled all the typing, and to Mrs Monique Boulet, who prepared the manuscripts for printing, but certainly also to the speakers and Workshop chairpersons, whose cooperation helped to make publication possible in such a short space of time.

Lucio Zichella
Malcolm Whitehead
Pieter van Keep

Keynote address

1

The neuropeptide concept and the menopause

D DE WIED AND TJ. B. VAN WIMERSMA GREIDANUS

Introduction

Neuropeptides are endogenous substances present in nerve cells and involved in nervous system function. Neuropeptides are formed in large proteins and several may arise in the same molecule such as adrenocorticotrophin (ACTH), β-lipotrophin (β-LPH), β-endorphin, etc., in pro-opiomelanocortin (POMC). A cascade of processes takes place in peptidergic neurons to express the genetic information as biologically active neuropeptides. These processes determine the quantities of neuropeptides synthesized and their biological activity through size, form and derivation. Transcription of a gene into precursor ribonucleic acid (RNA) is the initial step. Splicing of the precursor RNA results in formation of mature messenger RNA (mRNA). Alternative splicing patterns may generate different mRNAs from a single gene, resulting in different sets of neuropeptides. For example, calcitonin and calcitonin-gene-related peptide (CGRP) are derived from the same gene but are encoded by different mRNAs, depending on the cell in which the gene is expressed. In thyroid tissue the mRNA encodes calcitonin, thus affecting calcium metabolism, while in brain tissue it encodes CGRP, with vasodilative effects[1]. Different mRNAs from one gene control the production of substance P and the various tachykinins in a similar way[2,3].

Enzymatic processing of peptide precursors translated from mRNA forms sets of biologically active principles. While differential splicing of precursor RNA can be a cell-specific phenomenon, so can processing of neuropeptides from the same precursor as, for example, with pro-

3

opiomelanocortin (POMC). The anterior pituitary corticotrophs and the intermediate lobe melanotrophs convert POMC to different sets of peptides. The main products in the anterior lobe are β-LPH and ACTH, while part of β-LPH is further processed to γ-LPH and β-endorphin (βE-(1–31))[4]. In the intermediate lobe, ACTH is processed to α-melanocyte-stimulating hormone (α-MSH) and corticotrophin-like intermediate lobe peptide (CLIP) or ACTH-(18–39). More γ-LPH and βE-(1–31) is produced in this tissue than in the anterior pituitary. Both tissues produce γ-MSH related peptides from the 16-K N-terminal fragment[5]. The predominant peptides produced in brain tissue are α-MSH, ACTH fragments and βE-(1–31), but further processing to γ- and α-type endorphins also takes place.

POMC peptides undergo several non-proteolytic co-translational and post-translational modifications such as acetylation, sulphation, glycosylation and phosphorylation which may affect their biological activity. For example, N-acetylation of ACTH-(1–13) amide to α-MSH enhances the melanotrophic and behavioural effects[6]. Conversely, N-acetyl-γ-endorphin (Ac γE), which is the main form of γE in the intermediate lobe and in extrahypothalamic regions such as the septum, hippocampus and amygdala[7], eliminates the opioid activity but not the behavioural effect. Cholecystokinin-like peptides in the brain occur in the sulphated $Tyr^2(SO_3H)$ (CCK(S)) and non-sulphated CCK(NS) form. These peptides have neuroleptic-like activity in several of the test systems used for predicting antipsychotic activity. Effects on avoidance behaviour, grasping responses and interaction with the dopamine agonist apomorphine indicate that both the sulphated and the non-sulphated form exhibit such effects[8]. Only the sulphated form induces gall bladder contraction[9]. The sulphate group is not only important for peripheral action but also for the central effect. In contrast to CCK(NS), CCK(S) causes a decrease in locomotion following micro-injection into the nucleus accumbens[10]. Accordingly, cell-specific processing and derivation seem to be forms of neuropeptide plasticity by which neurotransmission can be modulated.

Neuroactive and neurotrophic effects of peptides derived from POMC

Numerous experiments with peptides related to ACTH/MSH involving tests such as avoidance, approach, discrimination and rewarded behaviour indicate that these peptides affect learning, motivation, attention, concentration and memory retrieval processes[11,12]. The peptides are also involved in grooming behaviour, stretching and yawning, and sexual behaviour[13]. The latter effects can be demonstrated only following intracranial injection. ACTH and related peptides possess in addition trophic effects on the nervous system, as shown in brain development[14] and nerve regeneration, and they also affect muscular performance[15,16]. In addition, these peptides modulate agonistic and social behaviour[17–19].

In the 16K fragment of POMC a peptide is found with a structure resembling that of α-MSH and β-MSH. The common core ACTH-(4–10) differs at the fifth place, which contains glycine instead of glutamine. Although its melanotrophic effect is minor and it has been termed γ-MSH, its behavioural activity is opposite to that of ACTH-(4–10) and related peptides. It is regarded as an endogenous opiate antagonist[20]. The N-terminal 16K fragment of POMC also has important trophic effects on the adrenal cortex[21,22].

The effect of ACTH on avoidance behaviour resides in the NH_2 terminal portion, since the tests showed ACTH-(4–10) to be as active as ACTH-(1–24), while ACTH-(11–24) possessed only slight activity. The tetrapeptide ACTH-(4–7) is the shortest active sequence to have essentially the same behavioural effect as ACTH[23], although more activity sites may be present. The residual behavioural potency observed for the sequence ACTH-(7–10) could be increased to the same level as that of the reference peptide ACTH-(4–10) by extending the C-terminal to ACTH-(7–16). Structure-activity studies with ACTH for other nervous system effects indicate different N-terminal moieties for a number of these effects.

There is evidence that ACTH generates such neuropeptides in the brain. ACTH-(1–39) is partially processed in the same way as was found for the intermediate lobe of the pituitary. Smaller fragments of this peptide, e.g. ACTH-(1–13)-NH_2, and the acetylated form of α-MSH are present in the brain. ACTH-(1–16), which carries almost all the nervous system effects, is one of the products of the conversion of ACTH-(1–39) by rat brain cell membranes *in vitro*[24]. Such *in vitro* studies indicate the capacity of the brain to form active fragments from large peptides.

If βE-(1–31) and related peptides are given intracranially in sufficient amounts they produce a variety of effects which are also induced by morphine and related compounds e.g. analgesia, respiratory depression, hypothermia, catatonia, exophtalmus, piloerection and loss of righting reflex. Fragments of βE-(1–31) or βE-(1–17) (γE) or βE-(1–16) (αE) are less active in this respect than the parent compound[12]. The endorphins also affect learned behaviour, but their effects are variable. Avoidance behaviour is blocked or facilitated by βE-(1–31) depending, on dose, time of administration and test procedure. When administered i.c.v. βE-(1–31) induces grooming which differs from that elicited by ACTH/MSH fragments and which is not associated with stretching, yawning or penile erection[13,25]. In contrast, it inhibits sexual behaviour[26]. The opiate-like effect of β-endorphin decreases following fragmentation of the peptide. However, fragmentation causes the generation of neuropeptides such as γ- and α-endorphins and related peptides with different central nervous system (CNS) effects[27]. It is known that βE-(1–17), (γE), facilitates extinction of active avoidance behaviour[28,29] and food-rewarded behaviour[29], enhances problem solving[30], delays extinction of a water-rewarded runway task[31], and attenuates passive avoidance behaviour[28]. The effect on avoidance behaviour is not dependent on opiate receptor activation, since the removal of the N-terminal amino acid residue, tyrosine, which eliminates opiate-like activity, enhances the influence of γ-endorphin on active and passive avoidance behaviour. Endorphins of the γ-type were found to possess neuroleptic-like effects. Arguments in favour are their influence on avoidance behaviour, their positive effects on the grasping response[28], the reduction in electrical self-stimulation elicited from the ventral tegmental area and nucleus accumbens at threshold currents[32,33], and their antagonistic influence on apomorphin-induced hypolocomotion[34]. Structure-activity studies revealed that βE-(6–17) is the shortest sequence with full neuroleptic-like activities. The Met-enkephalin moiety, which in itself has an effect opposite to that of γ-type endorphins[35], can be removed from γ-endorphin, while the neuroleptic-like activity persists.

It has been found that αE delays the extinction of pole-jumping avoidance behaviour and facilitates passive avoidance behaviour[28,35,36], delays the extinction of a food-rewarded response[29] and a water-rewarded runway task[31], and attenuates problem solving[30]. It also stimulates electrical self-stimulation at threshold currents in the ventral tegmental area but not in the nucleus accumbens[32,33]. It has been suggested that α-type endorphins produce effects which resemble those of psychostimulant drugs such as amphetamine[37,38]. In addition, αE and related peptides potentiate the increased activity induced by apomorphine and amphetamine[39,40]. Structure-activity studies on extinction of pole-jumping avoidance behaviour showed that while removal of the NH_2 terminal tyrosine residue does not affect the potency of αE, removal of the enkephalin moiety markedly reduces its effect[41]. In fact, the activity resides in βE-(2–9)[42]. Further studies demonstrated that αE potentiates stereotyped sniffing elicited by apomorphine, whereas γ-type endorphins do not interfere with this response[40]. The site of interaction of apomorphine and βE-(2–9) is presumably the nucleus caudatus, since local injection of both the drug and the peptide into that area, but not into the nucleus accumbens, induces effects similar to those found following peripheral treatment[40,42]. Other fragments of β-endorphin, such as βE-(10–16), may possess serotonin-like effects[43], or opioid antagonistic effects, as were found with βE-(1–27) and βE-(1–26)[44].

The neurohypophyseal hormones, vasopressin and oxytocin, and related peptides, modulate learning and memory processes. More recent studies discovered a multitude of central effects ranging from brain development to maternal behaviour, from thermoregulation to cardiovascular regulation, from sexual behaviour to drug-seeking behaviour[45].

Releasing hormones also possess CNS activity. Corticotrophin-releasing hormone (CRH) enhances neuronal activity in a variety of brain structures and stimulates sympathetic drive. It affects several types of behaviour, including locomotion, grooming rearing, food consumption and learned behaviour[46,47], and central administration of CRH results in a generalized activation of the sympatho-adrenomedullary system[48]. A central role for CRH in adaptation and in the neuroendocrine and autonomic responses to stress has been suggested[46,49,50].

Somatostatin has been shown to reduce locomotor activity and to increase stereotype behaviour in rats. It induces prolonged compulsive scratching, circulatory movements and sometimes barrel rotation, reduces slow-wave and rapid eye movement (REM) sleep and antagonizes electroconvulsive shock (ECS) induced amnesia in rats[51–53].

Thyrotrophin-releasing hormone (TRH) has been postulated to be an endogenous mediator in arousal behaviour, since administration of this neuropeptide results in locomotor and behavioural stimulatory effects[54]. TRH antagonizes sedation and hypothermia induced by barbiturates, ethanol and several other CNS depressants. It can reverse naturally-occurring CNS depression, i.e. sleep and hibernation. These analeptic effects of TRH have been observed in rats, mice, hamsters, gerbils, guinea-pigs and monkeys[52], and appear to occur independently of its classical endocrine actions. Despite these analeptic effects it has been suggested that TRH may function to stabilize the level of behavioural arousal, minimizing episodes of both hypo-activity and hyperactivity[51]. TRH produces dose-related decreases in food consumption and food-reinforced bar-press responses. It has a slight inhibitory effect on extinction of active avoidance behaviour. No effects on electrical self-stimulation have been observed. TRH also affects temperature and, depending on the animal species, hypothermia and hyperthermia have been reported[51,52]. Like TRH, luteinizing hormone releasing hormone (LH–RH) also limits sleep after sedative administration and reduces the duration of narcosis induced by pentobarbital. However, the most pronounced effect of LH–RH is its influence on sexual behaviour in female and male rats. In females it facilitates lordosis behaviour[55,56] and in intact males it reduces latency to intromission and ejaculation[57,58]. LH–RH also exerts effects on learned behaviour[59-61]. It enhances retention of active and passive avoidance behaviour. Moreover, LH–RH affects thermoregulation; it can raise or lower temperature, depending on species and site of administration[62,63]. Changes in cognitive functions have been reported following administration of LH–RH in men[64]. LH–RH appears to prevent improvement in a spatial orientation test relative to placebo condition, whereas its administration significantly increases performance in a fluency task. In addition, a significant lowering of plasma LH has been reported in depressed post-menopausal women as compared with post-menopausal controls[65]. Depression is usually associated with a reduction in cognitive functions[66]. These data point to changes in LH–RH in depressed post-menopausal women and to LH–RH effects on cognitive functions.

The study on the influence of the various neuropeptides related to ACTH, the endorphins and the neurohypophyseal hormones has so far revealed that these peptides affect motivation, attention, concentration (arousal), aggression, social behaviour, grooming behaviour, developmental processes, nerve cell regeneration, sexual behaviour, pain, addiction, mood, learning and memory processes, food intake, temperature regulation, and maternal behaviour. In addition, peptides related to β-endorphin appear to exert psychostimulant and neuroleptic-like effects, and peptides related to ACTH exhibit neurotrophic effects.

Congenital or acquired disturbances in neuropeptide systems may well be aetiological factors in psychiatric and neurological disorders. These disturbances might be caused by changes in the gene structure or gene expression, or the processing of precursor molecules, or their metabolism and their binding sites. These changes, in turn, may cause disturbances in the composition of neuropeptides or their biological effects.

Neuropeptide function, aging and menopause

Destruction of peptide-producing cells or disturbances in the production or processing of precursor molecules during development or aging and as a result of infection, trauma, alcohol and other toxic influences and stress, may be underlying causes of behavioural abnormalities. Aging is accompanied by degeneration of brain tissue and abnormal processing of neuropeptides. Aging causes cell loss in the human suprachiasmatic nucleus (SCN) in subjects 80 years of age and older[67]. This is more pronounced in patients suffering from Alzheimer's disease[68]. Post-translational changes may also occur in aging. The level of α-amidation activity in the CNS and cerebrospinal fluid (CSF) of patients with Alzheimer's disease is much lower than in control subjects[69]. Aging may affect other post-translational processing of neuropeptides as well. Wilkinson and Dorsa (1986)[70] found that more than 35% of γE in the hypothalamus of aged rats was in the acetylated form as against only 3% in adult animals. Aging also affects the neuropeptide concentration in the brain. It decreases immunoreactive βE, ACTH and α-MSH in rats[71-74]. The cerebral fluid concentration of vasopressin and somatostatin in patients with Alzheimer's disease is decreased, but that of βE and oxytocin is not[75-79]. A decrease in vasoactive intestinal polypeptide (VIP) in the brain has been demonstrated recently[80]. Interestingly, the number of type I hippocampal corticosterone receptors (CR), which is decreased in senescent rats, can be normalized by chronic treatment with the ACTH–(4–9) analogue Org 2766[81].

The cessation of reproductive function in the human female is related to a decline in ovarian function. It is possibly due to changes in the ovary and not to altered hypothalamic or pituitary function. The menopause is an irreversible result of aging, which starts at around 50 years of age. Loss of ovarian follicles and atrophy of the gland are the anatomical correlates. It is preceded by a rise in gonadotrophin secretion, mainly of follicle-stimulating hormone (FSH), while oestrogen production initially remains at a constant level and ovulation continues, albeit irregularly[82,83]. It has been suggested that an 'inhibin'-like substance which normally suppresses FSH secretion, and an age-related decrease in hypothalamic sensitivity to ovarian hormones play a role in this phenomenon. Higher doses of both oestrogen and testosterone appear necessary to suppress LH levels[84]. Circulating endogenous immunoreactive LH–RH becomes more frequently detectable[85] and LH–RH levels in the plasma of post-menopausal women seem to be elevated.

Besides the physical signs of the marked and relatively rapidly occurring change in hormonal activities, symptoms such as hot flushes, palpitations, headaches, muscular aches and other somatic disturbances, as well as depression, anxiety, cognitive effects (memory and concentration disturbances), are also characteristics of the climacteric syndrome. Several of these symptoms can be alleviated by chronic treatment with oestrogens[86,87]. Although the occurrence of hot flushes is an important feature of menopausal complaints, little is known about the exact mechanism underlying this phenomenon. Climacteric hot flushes appear to occur in close temporal proximity to the pulsatile release of LH. However, it has been suggested that hot flushes are not triggered by altered LH–RH secretion as such, but rather by altered afferent inputs to LH–RH neurons, which are secondary to hypogonadism[88].

Oestrogen therapy is effective in ameliorating or abolishing these episodes. The suggestion that gonadotrophin excess rather than oestrogen lack is responsible appears not to be true, since LH release can be temporarily blocked by short-term oestrogen treatment. Flushing episodes are not affected by such treatment[89]. Hot flushes, palpitations and headaches may also be related to increased levels of prolactin[90]. In addition, it is known that hypothalamic vasomotor function, which plays a role in flushing, is regulated in a feedback fashion by oestrogens.

However, there is evidence that substance P or opioid peptides also play a role in modulating vasomotor function. One out of a variety of LH–RH analogues which were developed as agonists or antagonists for putative LH–RH receptors regulating gonadotrophin release and reproduction has been found to inhibit the sympathetic vasomotor outflow. This LH–RH antagonist seems to be a substance-P-receptor antagonist in the CNS without peripheral effects[91].

Interestingly, the level of βE was found to be increased in women complaining of hot flushes and naloxone was able to reduce the frequency of hot flushes[92]. Conversely, βE and β-LPH are decreased in the menopause[93]. This decrease is associated with a decrease in pain threshold. Treatment with sex steroids, in particular with the progestational compound Org OD 14, raises this threshold as well as the levels of circulating βE and β-LPH[94]. Moreover, in the chronic absence of gonadal steroids in the post-menopause, the opiate-mediated control of gonadotrophin secretion disappears[95], while progestogens, at the doses used for the treatment of menopausal flushes, also increase endogenous opioid peptide activity, which restores opioid control of gonadotrophin secretion.

Thus, progestogen therapy may improve menopausal symptoms by a mechanism involving an increase in hypothalamic opiate activity[96], suggesting interactions between ovarian steroids, opioid peptides and LH–RH in the brain. In addition, it is interesting to note that hot flushes and mental symptoms are occasionally also observed in hypopituitarism. This may suggest that these complaints are not exclusively due to changes in the hypothalamic-pituitary-gonadal axis.

Thus, derangements in the cascade of processes might occur in peptidergic neurons. Cell-specific gene expression, cell-specific processing and cell-specific co-translational and post-translational modifications as a result of inborn errors or the destruction of peptide-producing cells due to trauma, aging, infections, toxic substances and stress may cause disturbances in brain functions. This may also hold for the menopause. Abnormalities, however minor, may affect feedback regulation and derange homeostatic control. Such disturbances may be factors in psychosomatic disorders. More studies are needed to substantiate these ideas. However, if they are correct, such disorders might eventually be amenable to treatment with the neuropeptides.

REFERENCES

1. Rosenfeld, M. G., Mermod, J. J., Amara, S. G. et al. (1983). Production of a novel neuropeptide encoded by the calcitonin-gene via tissue-specific RNA processing. *Nature*, **304**, 129
2. Nawa, H., Kotanie, H and Nakanishi, S. (1984). Tissue-specific generation

of two preprotachykinin mRNAs from one gene by alternative RNA splicing. *Nature*, **312**, 729

3. Nakanishi, S. (1985). Structure and regulation of the preprotachykinin gene. *Trends Neurosci.*, January, **41**

4. Eipper, B. A. and Mains, R. E. (1980). Structure and biosynthesis of pro-adreno-corticotrophin/endorphin and related peptides. *Endocrine Rev.*, **1**, 1

5. Pedersen, R. C., Ling, N. and Brownie, A. C. (1982). Immunoreactive γ-melanotropin in rat pituitary and plasma: a partial characterization. *Endocrinology*, **110**, 825

6. O'Donohue, T. L. and Dorsa, D. M. (1982). The opiomelanotropinergic neuronal and endocrine systems. *Peptides*, **3**, 353

7. Wiegant, V. M., Verhoef, J., Burbach, J. P. H. et al. (1985). N^{α}-acetyl-γ-endorphin is an endogenous non-opioid neuropeptide with biological activity. *Life Sci.*, **36**, 2277

8. Van Ree, J. M., Gaffori, O. and De Wied, D. (1983). In rats, the behavioural profile of CCK-8 related peptides resembles that of antipsychotic agents. *Eur. J. Pharmacol.*, **93**, 63

9. Van Ree, J. M. and De Wied, D. (1985). Neuroleptic-like activity and antipsychotic action of cholecystokinin-related peptides. *Ann. N.Y. Acad. Sci.*, **448**, 671

10. Fekete, M., Lengyel, A., Hegedüs, B. et al. (1984). Further analysis of the effects of cholecystokinin octapeptides on avoidance behaviour in rats. *Eur. J. Pharmacol.*, **98**, 79

11. Sandman, C. A. and Kastin, A. J. (1981). The influence of fragments of the LPH chains on learning, memory and attention in animals and man. *Pharmacol. Ther.*, **13**, 39

12. De Wied, D. and Jolles, J. (1982). Neuropeptides derived from proopiocortin: behavioural, physiological and neurochemical effects. *Physiol. Rev.*, **62**, 976

13. Gispen, W. H. and Isaacson, R. L. (1986). Excessive grooming in response to ACTH. In D. De Wied, W. H. Gispen and Tj. B. Van Wimersma Greidanus (eds.). *Neuropeptides and Behavior*, Vol. 1, pp. 273–312. (Oxford: Pergamon Press)

14. Swaab, D. F. and Martin, J. T. (1981). Functions of α-melanotropin and other opio-melanocortin peptides in labour, intrauterine growth and brain development. In D. Evered and G. Lawrenson (eds.). *Peptides of the Pars Intermedia*, Ciba Foundation Symposium 81, pp. 196–217. (London: Pitman Medical)

15. Strand, F. L. and Smith, C. M. (1986). LPH, ACTH, MSH and motor systems. In D. De Wied, W. H. Gispen and Tj. B. Van Wimersma Greidanus (eds.). *Neuropeptides and Behaviour*, Vol. 1, pp. 245–273. (Oxford: Pergamon Press)

16. Bijlsma, W. A., Schotman, P., Jennekens, F. G. I. et al. (1983). The enhanced recovery of sensorimotor function in rats is related to the melanotropic moiety of ACTH/MSH neuropeptides. *Eur. J. Pharmacol.*, **923**, 231

17. Leshner, A. I., Walker, W. A., Johnson, A. E. et al. (1973). Pituitary adrenocortical activity and intermale aggressiveness in isolated mice. *Physiol. Behav.*, **11**, 705

18. File, S. E. (1979). Effects of $ACTH_{4-10}$ in the social interaction tests of anxiety. *Brain Res.*, **171**, 157

19. Niesink, R. J. M. and Van Ree, J. M. (1984). Analysis of the facilitatory effect of the ACTH-(4–9) analog Org 2766 on active social contact in rats. *Life Sci.*, **34**, 961

20. Van Ree, J. M., Bohus, B., Csontos, K. M. et al. (1981). Behavioral profile of γ-MSH: relationship with ACTH and β-endorphin action. *Life Sci.*, **28**, 2875

21. Lowry, P. J., Silas, L., McLean et al. (1983). Pro-γ-melanocyte-stimulating hormone cleavage in adrenal gland undergoing compensatory growth. *Nature*, **306**, 70

22. Estivariz, F. E., Iturriza, F., McLean, C. et al. (1982). Stimulation of adrenal mitogenesis by N-terminal pro-opiocortin peptides. *Nature*, **297**, 419

23. Greven, H. M. and De Wied, D. (1977). Influence of peptides structurally related to ACTH and MSH on active avoidance behaviour in rats. A structure-activity relationship study. In F. J. H. Tilders, D. F. Swaab and Tj. B. van Wimersma Greidanus (eds.). *Melanocyte Stimulating Hormone: Control, Chemistry and Effects.* Frontiers of Hormone Research, Vol. 4, pp. 140–152. (Basel: Karger)

24. Wang, X.-C., Burbach, J. P. H. and Verhoef, J. (1983). Proteolysis of adrenocorticotropin in brain: characterization of cleavage sites by peptidases in synaptic membranes and formation of peptide fragment. *J. Biol. Chem.*, **258**, 7942

25. Van Wimersma Greidanus, Tj. B., Van de Brug, F., De Bruijckere, L. M. et al. (1987). Comparison of bombesin, ACTH and β-endorphin induced grooming: Antagonism by haloperidol, naloxone and neutrotensin. *N.Y. Acad. Sci.* (In press)

26. Meyerson, B. J. and Terenius, L. (1977). β-Endorphin and male sexual behaviour. *Eur. J. Pharmacol.*, **42**, 191

27. Burbach, J. P. H. (1986). Action of proteolytic enzymes on lipotropins and endorphins: biosynthesis, biotransformation and fate. In D. De Wied, W. H. Gispen, Tj. B. Van Wimersma Greidanus (eds.). *Neuropeptides and Behavior*, Vol. 1, pp. 43–76. (Oxford: Pergamon Press)

28. De Wied, D., Kovács, G. L., Bohus, B. et al. (1978). Neuroleptic activity of the neuropeptide β-LPH_{62-77} ([des-Tyr^1]) γ-endorphin; DTγE). *Eur. J. Pharmacol.*, **49**, 427

29. Koob, G. F., Le Moal, M. and Bloom, F. E. (1981). Enkephalin and endorphin influences on appetitive and aversive conditioning. In J. L. Martinez Jr., R. A. Jensen, R. B. Messing, H., Rigter and J. L. McGaugh (eds.). *Endogenous Peptides and Learning and Memory Processes*, pp. 249–267. (New York: Academic Press)

30. Bohus, B. (1980). Endorphins and behavioral adaptation. *Adv. Biol. Psychiatry*, **5**, 7

31. Le Moal, M., Koob, G. F. and Bloom, F. E. (1979). Endorphins in extinction: differential actions on appetitive and adversive tasks. *Life Sci.*, **24**, 1631

32. Dorsa, D. M., Van Ree, J. M. and De Wied, D. (1979). Effects of [Des-Tyr[1]]-γ-endorphin and α-endorphin on substantia nigra self-stimulation. *Pharmacol. Biochem. Behav.*, **10**, 899

33. Van Ree, J. M. and Otte, A. P. (1980). Effects of (Des-Tyr[1])-γ-endorphin and α-endorphin as compared to haloperidol and amphetamine on nucleus accumbens self-stimulation. *Neuropharmacology*, **29**, 429

34. Van Ree, J. M., Caffé, A. R. and Wolterink, G. (1982). Non-opiate β-endorphin fragments and dopamine. III. γ-Type endorphins and various neuroleptics counteract the hypoactivity elicited by intra-accumbens injection of apomorphine. *Neuropharmacology*, **21**, 1111

35. De Wied, D., Bohus, B., Van Ree, J. M. et al. (1978). Behavioral and electrophysiological effects of peptides related to lipotrophin (β-LPH). *J. Pharmacol. Exp. Ther.*, **204**, 570

36. Kovács, G. L. and De Wied, D. (1981). Endorphin influences on learning and memory. In J. L. Martinez Jr., R. A. Jensen, R. B. Messing, H. Rigter and J. L. McGaugh (eds.). *Endogenous Peptides and Learning and Memory Processes*, pp. 231–247. (New York: Academic Press)

37. De Wied, D. (1978). Psychopathology as a neuropeptide dysfunction. In J. M. van Ree and L. Terenius (eds.). *Characteristics and Function of Opioids*, pp. 113–122. (Amsterdam: Elsevier/North-Holland Biomedical Press)

38. Van Ree, J. M., Bohus, B. and De Wied, D. (1980). Similarity between behavioral effects of des-tyrosine-γ-endorphin and haloperidol and of α-endorphin and amphetamine. In E. Leong Way (ed.). *Endogenous and Exogenous Opiate Agonists and Antagonists*, pp. 459–462. (New York: Pergamon Press)

39. Kameyama, T. and Ukai, M. (1981). Multi-dimensional analyses of behaviour in mice treated with α-endorphin. *Neuropharmacology*, **20**, 247

40. Van Ree, J. M. (1982). Non-opiate β-endorphin fragments and dopamine. II. β-endorphin 2–9 enhances apomorphine-induced stereotypy following subcutaneous and intrastriatal injection. *Neuropharmacology*, **21**, 1103

41. Greven, H. M. and De Wied, D. (1980). Structure and behavioural activity of peptides related to corticotropin and lipotropin. In D. De Wied and P. A. van Keep, (eds.). *Hormones and the Brain*, pp. 115–127. (Lancaster: MTP Press)

42. Van Ree, J. M. and De Wied, D. (1982). Behavioural effects of the β-endorphin fragment 2–9. *Life Sci.*, **31**, 2383

43. Gaffori, O. and Van Ree, J. M. (1985). β-Endorphin-(10–16) antagonizes behavioural responses elicited by melatonin following injection into the nucleus accumbens of rats. *Life Sci.*, **37**, 357

44. Hammonds, R. G. Jr., Nicolas, P., Li, C. H. (1984). βE-(1–27) is an antagonist of β-endorphin analgesia. *Proc. Natl. Acad. Sci. USA*, **81**, 1389

45. De Wied, D. (1978). Neurohypophyseal hormone influences on learning

and memory processes. In G. Lynch, J. L. McGaugh and N. M. Weinberger (eds.). *Neurobiology of Learning and Memory*, pp. 289–312. (New York: Guilford Press)

46. Fekete, M., Szántó-Fekete, M. and Telegdy, G. (1987). Action of corticotropin-releasing factor on the nervous system. In G. Telegdy (ed.). *Neuropeptides and Brain Function*, Frontiers of Hormone Research, Vol. 15. (Basel: Karger) (In press)

47. Veldhuis, H. D. and De Wied, D. (1984). Differential behavioural actions of corticotropin-releasing factor (CRF). *Pharmacol. Biochem. Behav.*, **21**, 707

48. Brown, M. R., Fisher, L. A., Spiess, J. et al. (1982). Corticotropin-releasing factor: action on the sympathetic nervous system and metabolism. *Endocrinology*, **111**, 928

49. Tilders, F. J. H. and Berkenbosch, F. (1986). CRF and catecholamines; their place in the central and peripheral regulation of the stress response. *Acta Endocrinol.*, **112**, (Suppl.), 276, 63

50. Swanson, L. W., Sawchenko, P. E., Rivier, J. et al. (1983). Organisation of ovine corticotropin-releasing factor immunoreactive cells and fibers in the rat brain, an immunohistochemical study. *Neuroendocrinology*, **36**, 165

51. Nemeroff, C. B., Kalivas, P. W., Golden, R. N. et al. (1984). Behavioural effects of hypothalamic hypophysiotropic hormones, neurotensin, substance P and other neuropeptides. *Pharmacol. Ther.*, **24**, 1

52. Prange, A. J., Nemeroff, Ch. B. and Loosen, P. T. (1978). Behavioural effects of hypothalamic peptides. In J. Hughes (ed.). *Centrally Acting Peptides*, pp. 99–118. (London: McMillan Press Ltd.)

53. Vécsei, L., Balasz, M. and Telegdy, G. (1987). Action of somatostatin on the central nervous system. In G. Telegdy (ed.). *Neuropeptides and Brain Function*, Frontiers of Hormone Research, Vol. 15. (Basel: Karger) (In press)

54. Reichlin, S. (1986). Neural functions of TRH. *Acta Endocrinol.*, **112**, (Suppl.), 276, 21

55. Moss, R. L. and McCann, S. M. (1973). Induction of mating behaviour in rats by luteinizing hormone-releasing factor. *Science*, **181**, 177

56. Pfaff, D. W. (1973). Luteinizing hormone-releasing factor potentiates lordosis behaviour in hypophysectomized ovariectomized female rats. *Science*, **182**, 1148

57. Moss, R. L., McCann, S. M. and Dudley, C. A. (1975). Releasing hormones in sexual behaviour. *Progr. Brain Res.*, **42**, 37

58. Moss, R. L. and Foreman, M. M. (1976). Potentiation of lordosis behaviour by intrahypothalamic infusion of synthetic luteinizing hormone-releasing hormone. *Neuroendrocrinology*, **20**, 176

59. De Wied, D., Witter, A. and Greven, H. M. (1975). Behaviourally active ACTH analogues. *Biochem. Pharmacol.*, **24**, 1463

60. Mora, S. and Diaz Veliz, G. (1983). Influence of luteinizing hormone releasing hormone (LHRH) on the behavioural effects of amphetamine in rats. *Pharmacol. Biochem. Behav.*, **19/2**, 157

61. Mora, S. and Diaz Veliz, G. (1985). Luteinizing-hormone-releasing hormone modifies retention of passive and active avoidance responses in rats. *Psychopharmacology*, **85/3**, 315

62. Nemeroff, C. B., Osbahr, A. J. III, Manberg, P. J. et al. (1979). Alterations in nociception and body temperature after intracisternally administered neurotensin, β-endorphin, other endogenous peptides, and morphine. *Proc. Natl. Acad. Sci. USA*, **76**, 5368

63. Lomax, P., Bajorek, J. G., Chesanek, W. et al. (1980). Thermoregulatory effects of luteinizing hormone-releasing hormone in the rat. In B. Cox, P. Lomax, A. S. Milton and E. Schönbaum (eds.). *Thermoregulatory Mechanisms and Their Therapeutic Implications*, pp. 208–211. (Basel: Karger)

64. Gordon, H. W., Corbin, E. D. and Lal, P. A. (1986). Changes in specialized cognitive function following changes in hormone levels. *Cortex*, **22/3**, 399

65. Sachar, E. J. (1975). Neuroendocrine abnormalities in depressive illness. In E. J. Sachar (ed.). *Topics in Psychoendocrinology*, pp. 135–156. (New York: Grune and Stratton)

66. Cohen, R. M., Weingartner, H. Smallberg, S. A. et al. (1982). Effort and cognition in depression. *Arch. Gen. Psychiat.*, **39**, 593

67. Swaab, D. F., Fliers, E. and Partiman, T. S. (1985). The suprachiasmatic nucleus of the human brain in relation to sex, age and senile dementia. *Brain Res.*, **342**, 37

68. Swaab, D. F. and Fliers, E. (1985). A sexually dimorphic nucleus in the human brain. *Science*, **228**, 1112

69. Wand, G. S., May, C., May, V. et al. (1986). Peptide alpha-amidation activity is low in the central nervous systems (CSF) of patients with Alzheimer's disease. Abstracts *68th Ann. Meeting Endocrine Soc.*, p. 288, Anaheim, USA

70. Wilkinson, C. W. and Dorsa, D. M. (1986). The effects of aging on molecular forms of beta- and gamma-endorphins in rat hypothalamus. *Neuroendocrinology*, **43**, 124

71. Barden, N., Dupont, A., Labrie, F. et al. (1981). Age-dependent changes in the β-endorphin content of discrete brain nuclei. *Brain Res.*, **208**, 209

72. Barnea, A., Cho, G. and Porter, J. C. (1982). A reduction in the concentration of immunoreactive corticotropin melanotropin and lipotropin in the brain of the aging rat. *Brain Res.*, **232**, 345

73. Dorsa, D. M., Smith, E. R. and Davidson, J. M. (1984). Immunoreactive β-endorphin and LHRH levels in the brains of aged male rats with impaired sex behaviour. *Neurobiol. Aging*, **5**, 115

74. Gambert, S. R., Garthwaite, T. L., Pontzer, C. H. et al. (1980). Age-related changes in central nervous system beta-endorphin and ACTH. *Neuroendocrinology*, **31**, 252

75. Raskind, M. A., Peskind, E. R., Lampe, T. H. et al. (1986). Cerebrospinal fluid vasopressin, oxytocin, somatostatin, and β-endorphin in Alzheimer's disease. *Arch. Gen. Psychiatry*, **43**, 382

76. Rossor, M. N., Iversen, L. L., Reynolds, G. P. et al. (1984). Neurochemical characteristics of early and late onset types of Alzheimer's disease. *Br. Med. J.*, **288**, 961

77. Ferrier, I. N., Cross, A. J., Johnson, J. A. et al. (1983). Neuropeptides in Alzheimer-type dementia. *J. Neurol. Sci.*, **62**, 159

78. Davies, P., Katzman, R. and Terry, R. D. (1980). Reduced somatostatin-like immuno-reactivity in cerebral cortex from cases of Alzheimer disease and Alzheimer senile dementia. *Nature*, **288**, 279

79. Wood, P. L., Etienne, P., Lal, S. et al. (1982). Reduced lumbar CSF somatostatin level in Alzheimer's disease. *Life Sci.*, **31**, 2073

80. Nakamura, K., Kaneko, H., Hayashi, M. et al. (1986). Vasoactive intestinal polypeptide (VIP) in human cerebrospinal fluid of dementia with cerebral atrophy. Abstracts *1st Int. Congress of Neuroendocrinology*, July 9–11, nr 331, San Francisco, USA

81. Reul, J. M. H. M., Tonnaer, J. A. D. M. and De Kloet, E. R. (1986). Selective increases of type I corticosteroid receptors in hippocampus of senescent rats after chronic treatment with a behaviourally potent ACTH-(4–9) analog. Abstracts *1st. Int. Congress of Neuroendocrinology*, July 9–11, nr 313, San Francisco, USA

82. Sherman, B. M., West, J. H. and Korenman, S. G. (1976). The menopausal transition: analysis of LH, FSH, estradiol and progesterone concentrations during menstrual cycles of older women. *J. Clin. Endocrinol.*, **42**, 629

83. Reyes, F. I., Winter, J. S. D. and Faiman, Ch. (1977). Pituitary-ovarian relationships preceding the menopause. I. A cross-sectional study of serum follicle-stimulating hormone, luteinizing hormone, prolactin, estradiol, and progesterone levels. *Am. J. Obstet. Gynecol.*, **129**, 557

84. Muta, K., Kato, K., Akamine, Y. et al. (1980). Age-related changes in feedback regulation of gonadotropin secretion by sex steroids in men. *6th Int. Congress of Endocrinology*, February 10–16, Abstract 257, Melbourne, Australia

85. Mortimer, C. H. (1977). Gonadotropin-Releasing Hormone. In L. Martini and G. M. Besser (eds.). *Clinical Neuroendocrinology*, pp. 213–236. (New York: Academic Press)

86. Lobo, R. A., Cristo, M. and Crary, W. (1987). Effects of estrogen on psychological function in asymptomatic post-menopausal women. *5th International Congress on the Menopause*, April 1987, Abstract nr. 66, Sorrento, Italy

87. Montgomery, J. C., Appleby, L. and Studd, J. W. W. (1987). Placebo-controlled study of the response of psychiatric disturbances at the menopause to oestradiol and oestradiol/testosterone implants. *5th International Congress on the Menopause*, April 1987, Abstract nr. 111, Sorrento, Italy

88. Gambone, J., Meldrum, D. R., Laufer, L. et al. (1984). Further delineation of hypothalamic dysfunction responsible for menopausal hot flushes. *J. Clin. Endocrinol. Metab.*, **59**, 1097

89. Casper, R. F. (1979). Physical, neuroendocrine and neuropharmacologic

correlates during menopausal flushes. *61st Ann. Meeting Endocrine Society*, Abstract 210

90. Koyama, T., Ichimura, M., Ohara, M. et al. (1987). Computerized analysis of correlations between climacteric symptoms and serum levels of oestradiol, prolactin, testosterone and cortisol. *5th International Congress on the Menopause*, April 1987, Abstract nr. 183, Sorrento, Italy

91. Takano, Y., Sawyer, W. B., Sanders, N. L. et al. (1985). LH–RH analogue act as Substance P. antagonist by inhibiting spinal cord vasomotor responses. *Brain Res.*, **337**, 357

92. Schurz, B., Metka, M., Kurz, K. et al. (1987). β-Endorphin in climacteric women. *5th International Congress on the Menopause*, April 1987, Abstract nr. 210, Sorrento, Italy

93. Facchinetti, F., Alfonsi, E., Golinelli, S. et al. (1987). Effects of post-menopausal therapies on pain perception. *5th International Congress on the Menopause*, April 1987, Abstract nr. 84, Sorrento, Italy

94. Facchinetti, F., Golinelli, S., Campanini, D. et al. (1987). Response of plasma β-endorphin (β-EP) and β-lipotrophin (β-LPH) to clonidine, 5-hydroxytryptophane, and domperidone in post-menopausal women treated with Org OD14 or oestradiol valerate. *5th International Congress on the Menopause*, April 1987, Abstract nr. 188, Sorrento, Italy

95. Reid, R. L., Quigley, M. R. and Yen, S. S. C. (1983). The disappearance of opioidergic regulation of gonadotropin secretion in postmenopausal women. *J. Clin. Endocrinol. Metab.*, **57**, 1107

96. Casper, R. F., Alapin-Rubillovitz, S. (1985). Progestins increase endogenous opioid peptide activity in postmenopausal women. *J. Clin. Endocrinol. Metab.*, **60**, 34

SECTION 1

Plenary lectures

2

Cancer of the breast in relation to hormone therapy in the peri-menopause and post-menopause

M. P. VESSEY

Introduction

Age at menarche, age at first full-term pregnancy and age at natural or artificial menopause all exert important influences on the risk of breast cancer. Although the precise way in which these factors act is not known, it seems certain that hormonal mechanisms are involved. Accordingly, it is entirely plausible that administered hormones should also affect breast cancer risk. The relevant epidemiological literature is reviewed here with special reference to replacement therapy in peri-menopausal and post-menopausal women.

Administration of hormones during pregnancy and for contraception

There is reasonably convincing evidence that women who were given stilboestrol in large doses during pregnancy suffered a modest increase in the risk of breast cancer some 20 years later[1], but this observation is of doubtful relevance to the prolonged use of low doses of oestrogens (with or without progestogens) by menopausal women. Combined oral contraceptives seem to have no effect at all on breast cancer risk when used by women in the middle of reproductive life (i.e. broadly between the ages of 25 and 39 years), even if they are taken for many years[2]. Controversy still rages, however, about the possible adverse effects of combined oral contraceptives on breast cancer risk when they are taken for long periods at a very early age[3] or before the first full-term pregnancy[4]. But here again, whatever the truth may be, the relevance to hormone replacement (if any) is far from obvious. Limited data are also available concerning the effects on the breast of depot-medroxy progesterone acetate (Depo-Provera) used as a contraceptive. The latest figures from the World Health Organization Study[5] suggest that the risk of cancer is neither increased nor decreased by such treatment, but further data are awaited from Lee's study in Costa Rica and Skegg's study in New Zealand.

Administration of hormones around the time of the menopause

Results are now available from a substantial number of epidemiological studies directly concerned with the relationship between hormone use in peri-menopausal and post-menopausal women and breast cancer risk. Early studies, of both the case-control and the cohort type, had too many shortcomings to be of much value, but for what they are worth, they did not suggest any increase in risk[6]. The first study to approach modern epidemiological research standards concerned 1,891 women in Louisville, Kentucky, who had been given long-term treatment with conjugated oestrogens and followed up for an average of 12 years[7]. In total, 49 cases of breast cancer were observed, whereas 39 would have been expected on the basis of rates in the general population. The relative risk increased with follow-up duration, rising to 2.0 after 15 years. In addition, after 10 years of follow-up, two factors normally related to a low risk of breast cancer—multiparity and oophorectomy—no longer imparted a protective effect.

Most of the remaining recent studies have been of the case-control type. As Table 2.1 shows, all such studies have been conducted in the USA. This is not because epidemiologists elsewhere have no interest in the problem; rather it reflects the fact that the opportunities for research on hormone replacement therapy are particularly good in the USA, where such treatment has been widely used on a long-term basis. It should also be noted that by far the most common drug used by the women in each of the studies listed in Table 2.1[8-17] was Premarin (conjugated equine oestrogens).

Table 2.2 attempts to summarise the overall results of the 10 case-control studies indicating also, where possible, if the risk varied according to whether or not the women had intact ovaries. In general, the findings give little cause for concern, although some studies do suggest a modest elevation of risk, especially among women retaining

Table 2.1 RECENT CASE-CONTROL STUDIES OF HORMONE REPLACEMENT THERAPY AND BREAST CANCER

Reference	No. of cases	Source of cases
Ross et al. (1980)[8]	138	Two retirement communities in Los Angeles.
Jick et al. (1980)[9]	97	Group Health Cooperative, Puget Sound, Seattle.
Hoover et al. (1981)[10]	345	KFHP (health plan) Portland, Oregon.
Kelsey et al. (1981)[11]	332	Connecticut hospitals.
Hulka et al. (1982)[12]	199	N. Carolina hospitals.
Sherman et al. (1983)[13]	113	Iowa hospitals.
Kaufman et al. (1984)[14]	925	Many hospitals in USA and Canada.
Nomura et al. (1986)[15]	344	Hawaiian hospitals.
Brinton et al. (1986)[16]	1,960	Breast Cancer Detection Demonstration Project.
Wingo et al. (1987)[17]	1,369	Cancer and Steroid Hormone Study (all women under 55 years of age).

at least one ovary. Table 2.3 considers the effects of duration of use and medication dosage (the figures given all relate to Premarin). The provision of a concise summary of the data is difficult because different authors have analyzed their studies in different ways. Nonetheless, there is some indication that risk might increase with duration of use, but there is little evidence that dosage is important.

Particular attention must be given to the study by Brinton et al.[16], which is the biggest, covers a wide age range, includes large numbers of long-term users of replacement therapy, is one of the best conducted, and is certainly the most comprehensively analyzed. As indicated in Table 2.1, the subjects in this investigation participated in the Breast Cancer Detection Demonstration Project (BCDDP), a multicentre breast cancer screening programme involving over 280,000 women at 29 centres. Cases were those identified during the screening programme. Controls (matched for centre, race, age, time of entry to

Table 2.2 RECENT CASE-CONTROL STUDIES OF HORMONE REPLACEMENT THERAPY AND BREAST CANCER—OVERALL FINDINGS

Reference	Overall	*Relative risk in users:* One or more ovaries intact	Ovaries removed
Ross et al. (1980)[8]	1.1	1.4	0.8
Jick et al. (1980)[9]*	Not stated	3.4+	1.1
Hoover et al. (1981)[10]	1.4+	1.3	1.5
Kelsey et al. (1981)[11]	0.9	0.9	0.9
Hulka et al. (1982)[12]**	Not stated	1.7+ 1.8+	1.2 1.3
Sherman et al. (1983)[13]	0.6	Not stated	Not stated
Kaufman et al. (1984)[14]	0.8	0.9	0.5+
Nomura et al. (1986)[15]***	0.9 1.1	Not stated Not stated	Not stated Not stated
Brinton et al. (1986)[16]	1.0	1.0	1.1
Wingo et al. (1987)[17]	1.0	1.0	1.3

+   Relative risk differs significantly from 1.0.
*   Data analyzed according to hysterectomy status, not ovarian status.
** First row: comparison with hospital controls.
    Second row: comparison with community controls.
*** First row: Caucasian cases, community controls.
    Second row: Japanese cases, community controls.

the programme and length of continuation in the programme) were chosen from among women who had not been referred for biopsy during the course of screening participation. Data on hormone use and other matters were obtained at home interviews, which were successfully completed for 80% of eligible cases and 83% of controls.

As Table 2.3 indicates, this study has provided some evidence for an association between duration of hormone use and breast cancer risk. More comprehensive data are provided in Table 2.4, where it can be seen that the duration of use association is apparent, irrespective of type of menopause.

Other important findings in the study by Brinton et al.[16] include evidence for an increase in breast cancer risk in association with

Table 2.3 RECENT CASE-CONTROL STUDIES OF HORMONE REPLACEMENT THER-APY AND BREAST CANCER—EFFECT OF DURATION OF USE AND DOSE

	Positive association with:	
Reference	*Duration of use*	*Dose*
Ross et al. (1980)[8]	Positive relation with 'mg-months' of use in those with intact ovaries[(+)]	
Jick et al. (1980)[9]	No.	No.
Hoover et al. (1981)[10]*	Yes. ≥ 5 years, RR 1.7[(+)]	Yes. ≥ 1.25 mg, RR 1.8[(+)]
Kelsey et al. (1981)[11]	No relation with 'mg-months' of use, irrespective of ovarian status	
Hulka et al. (1982)[12]**	No. Ovaries intact ≥ 10 years, RR 0.7 ≥ 10 years, RR 1.7	No. Ovaries intact > 0.625 mg, RR 0.8 > 0.625 mg, RR 1.0
Sherman et al. (1983)[13]	No. No details given.	Not stated.
Kaufman et al. (1984)[14]***	Doubtful. ≥ 10 years, RR 1.3 ≥ 10 years, RR 0.5	No. ≥ 1.25 mg, RR 0.7 ≥ 1.25 mg, RR 0.5
Nomura et al. (1986)[15]****	Yes. > 6 years, RR 1.3 > 6 years, RR 1.9	Not stated.
Brinton et al. (1986)[16]*	Yes. ≥ 20 years, RR 1.5[(+)]	No. 2.5 mg, RR 0.8*****
Wingo et al. (1987)[17]	Yes ≥ 20 years, RR 1.8	Not stated

*	Controlled for type of menopause.
**	First row: comparison with hospital controls.
	Second row: comparison with community controls.
***	First row: ovaries intact.
	Second row: ovaries removed.
****	First row: Caucasian cases, community controls.
	Second row: Japanese cases, community controls.
*****	Preparation used longest.
+	Trend statistically significant.
RR	Relative risk.

Table 2.4 RELATIVE RISK OF BREAST CANCER IN RELATION TO DURATION OF
MENOPAUSAL HORMONE USE (MODIFIED FROM BRINTON ET AL. 1986,[16])

Duration of hormone use (years)	Natural menopause	Surgical menopause —ovaries retained	Relative risk: Surgical menopause —ovaries removed	Total
5	0.95	0.82	0.98	0.89 (0.8–1.0)
5–9	1.05	1.15	1.18	1.09 (0.9–1.3)
10–14	1.30	1.16	1.64	1.28 (0.9–1.6)
15–19	1.70	1.26	1.43	1.24 (0.9–1.8)
20				1.47 (0.9–2.3)
Trend test	$P = 0.03$	$P = 0.11$	$P = 0.03$	$P < 0.01$

long-term use of stilboestrol as well as Premarin and evidence that
women initiating hormone use subsequent to a diagnosis of benign
breast disease are at special risk. It is also of interest that the
hormone-breast cancer association was observed predominantly among
women with tumours in the more favourable stages, this situation
being similar to that repeatedly found for endometrial cancer.

In addition to the case-control studies, data have also been reported
recently from three cohort studies. Thomas et al.[18] followed up a
group of 1,439 women who were initially treated for biopsy-proven
benign breast disease between 1942 and 1975. Exogenous oestrogen
taken before the initial benign lesion was unrelated to breast cancer
risk. Subsequent use, however, eliminated the protective effect of
artificial menopause and appeared to act synergistically with epithelial
hyperplasia, papillomatosis and calcification in the original lesion to
increase breast cancer risk. Gambrell et al.[19] studied 5,563 post-
menopausal women at Wilford Hall USAF Medical Center and followed them up for a total of 37,236 person-years of observation. A
total of 53 women were found to have developed breast cancer. The
incidence in oestrogen users was not significantly different from that
expected from NCI SEER data, but there was evidence of a reduced
incidence in women using oestrogens and progestogens (8 cases
observed, relative risk 0.3, 95% confidence interval 0.1–0.8). However, the data are clearly insufficient to enable firm conclusions to be
drawn from this study. In addition, the published report provides little

information on how completely the women were followed up or how comparable the women were in the different groups which were contrasted. Most recently, Hunt et al.[20] have reported the preliminary results of a cohort study of 4,544 British women receiving replacement therapy. Many different preparations were used and about 43% of all use was 'opposed' by progestogens. In general, however, both the amount of progestogen and the number of days per cycle for which it was given were less than would have been the case if the women had been receiving modern opposed therapy. The findings in regard to breast cancer mortality were entirely reassuring; 12 deaths were observed, whereas 21.9 were expected on the basis of national rates (relative risk 0.55, 95% confidence interval 0.28–0.96). However, the cancer incidence results were less reassuring. In total, 50 women were found to have developed breast cancer during follow-up as against the 31.38 expected from cancer registry rates (relative risk 1.59, 95% confidence interval 1.18–2.10). Furthermore, there was no evidence in this study that oophorectomy imparted any protective effect (indeed, the reverse appeared to be true), while there was an indication of an increasing risk with duration of hormone use. There were no obvious differences in risk with type of therapy (i.e. unopposed versus opposed), but the use of unopposed ethinyloestradiol in particular appeared to have undesirable effects on the breast.

Comment

On balance, the available epidemiological literature suggests that prolonged use of oestrogens by peri-menopausal and post-menopausal women may slightly increase the risk of breast cancer and that this risk may be accentuated in women with pre-existing benign breast disease. Having said this, the possibility remains that at least some of the excess risk is attributable to more complete diagnosis of breast cancer in women using oestrogens than in other women. This point of view is supported by the favourable staging distribution of breast cancers in oestrogen users reported by Brinton et al.[16] and Hunt et al.[20].

It should be stressed that almost all the work published so far concerns the use of conjugated equine oestrogens; sadly almost nothing is known about the effects of products containing both an oestrogen and a progestogen. Furthermore, it may be many years yet before conclusive data become available on the forms of therapy now most commonly administered to women with intact uteri. The findings of Brinton et al.[16] suggest that follow-up for 10 or even 20 years is required.

Finally, on theoretical grounds, we should not perhaps be surprised if replacement therapy does have some small effect on breast cancer risk. In this context, it is helpful to consider the protective effect that early menopause offers. Pike et al.[21] have reported data from various studies which suggest that, for every 5 years menopause is delayed, there may be an approximately 33% increase in subsequent breast cancer risk. This implies that a 15-year difference in age at menopause might be associated with a twofold increase in risk. If the administration of replacement therapy can in any way be regarded as maintaining a woman in a pre-menopausal state, then findings such as those reported by Brinton et al. (1986) should not surprise us. By the same token, they should not unduly alarm us either, bearing in mind the age at which replacement therapy is usually commenced, the likely duration of therapy in most women and the favourable effects of treatment on bone and, most probably, on the cardiovascular system also. Furthermore, it is to be expected that replacement therapy will continue to become more and more finely tuned to minimize risks and maximize benefits.

REFERENCES

1. Greenberg, E. R., Barnes, A. B., Resseguie, L. et al. (1984). Breast cancer in mothers given diethylstilboestrol in pregnancy. *New Engl. J. Med.*, **311**, 1393
2. Vessey, M. P. (1985). Exogenous hormones. In M. P. Vessey, M. Gray (eds.). *Cancer: Risks and Prevention*, pp. 166–194. (Oxford: Oxford University Press)
3. Pike, M. C., Henderson, B. E., Casagrande, J. T. et al. (1981). Oral contraceptive use and early abortion as risk factors for breast cancer in young women. *Br. J. Cancer*, **43**, 72
4. McPherson, K., Neil, A., Vessey, M. P. et al. (1983). Oral contraceptives and breast cancer. *Lancet*, **ii**, 1414
5. World Health Organization. (1986). Depot-medroxyprogesterone acetate (DMPA) and cancer: Memorandum from a WHO meeting. *Bull. Wld. Hlth. Org.*, **64**, 375
6. Wynder, E. L., Schneiderman, M. A. (1973). Exogenous hormones—boon or culprit? *J. Natl. Cancer Inst.*, **51**, 729

7. Hoover, R., Gray, L. A., Cole, P. et al. (1976). Menopausal estrogens and breast cancer. *New Engl. J. Med.*, **295**, 401

8. Ross, R. K., Paganini-Hill, A., Gerkins, V. R. et al. (1980). A case-control study of menopausal estrogen therapy and breast cancer. *J. Amer. Med. Assoc.*, **243**, 1635

9. Jick, H., Walker, A. M., Watkins, R. N. et al. (1980). Replacement estrogens and breast cancer. *Amer. J. Epidemiol.*, **112**, 586

10. Hoover, R., Glass, A., Finkle, W. D. et al. (1981). Conjugated estrogens and breast cancer risk in women. *J. Natl. Cancer Inst.*, **67**, 815

11. Kelsey, J. L., Fischer, D. B., Holford, T. R. et al. (1981). Exogenous estrogens and other factors in the epidemiology of breast cancer. *J. Natl. Cancer Inst.*, **67**, 327

12. Hulka, B., Chambless, L. E., Deubner, D. C. et al. (1982). Breast cancer and estrogen replacement therapy. *Amer. J. Obstet. Gynecol.*, **143**, 638

13. Sherman, B., Wallace, R., Bean, J. (1983). Estrogen use and breast cancer: interaction with body mass. *Cancer*, **51**, 1527

14. Kaufman, D. W., Miller, D. R., Rosenberg, L. et al. (1984). Non contraceptive estrogen use and the risk of breast cancer. *J. Amer. Med. Assoc.*, **252**, 63

15. Nomura, A. M. Y., Kolonel, L. N., Hirohata, T. et al. (1986). The association of replacement estrogens with breast cancer. *Int. J. Cancer*, **37**, 49

16. Brinton, L. A., Hoover, R., Fraumeni, J. F. (1986). Menopausal oestrogens and breast cancer risk: an expanded case-control study. *Br. J. Cancer*, **54**, 825

17. Wingo, P. A., Layde, P. M., Lee, N. C. et al. (1987). The risk of breast cancer in postmenopausal women who have used estrogen replacement therapy. *J. Amer. Med. Assoc.*, **257**, 209

18. Thomas, D. B., Persing, J. P., Hutchinson, W. B. (1982). Exogenous estrogens and other risk factors for breast cancer in women with benign breast diseases. *J. Natl. Cancer Inst.*, **69**, 1017

19. Gambrell, R. D., Maier, R. C., Sanders, B. I. (1983). Decreased incidence of breast cancer in postmenopausal estrogen-progestogen users. *Obstet. Gynecol.*, **62**, 435

20. Hunt, K., Vessey, M., McPherson, K. et al. (1987). Long term surveillance of mortality and cancer incidence in women receiving hormone replacement therapy. *Br. J. Obstet. Gynaecol.*, **94**, 620

21. Pike, M. C., Henderson, B. E., Casagrande, J. T. (1981). The epidemiology of breast cancer as it relates to menarche, pregnancy and menopause. In Pike, M. C., Siiteri, P. K., Welsh, C. N. (eds.). *Banbury Report No. 8. Hormones and breast cancer.* Cold Spring Harbor Laboratory, 3

3

Exogenous oestrogens and ovarian cancer risk

D. W. CRAMER

Introduction

In this paper, the epidemiological associations between ovarian cancer and exogenous oestrogen, including menopausal hormones, will be considered. In addition, mechanisms which may possibly underlie such associations will be discussed.

It is by no means immediately obvious that there should be an association between exogenous oestrogen and ovarian cancer. Is it reasonable that an organ which itself produces oestrogen should be a target for the latter's mitogenic effects? That this association is biologically plausible is suggested by two observations. Firstly, oestrogen receptors are found in a majority of ovarian neoplasms[1,2] and, secondly, the most common types of ovarian cancer, the 'epithelial' tumours, have the appearance of müllerian structures which are known to be oestrogen-sensitive. Serous tumours of the ovary look like the epithelium lining the fallopian tubes, endometrioid tumours look like the endometrium, and mucinous tumours look like the endocervix.

Exogenous oestrogen – epidemiological evidence

If, then, there is a reasonable possibility that exogenous oestrogens might be related to ovarian cancer, what epidemiological data are available regarding this association? Descriptive epidemiological studies provide some evidence. In the early 1970s, a large increase occurred in the incidence of endometrial cancers in the United States, mostly in women aged 50–70[3]. This increase in incidence was correlated with an

31

increase in menopausal oestrogen sales, while a decrease in incidence followed a decrease in menopausal oestrogen sales. Over this same period, however, no major changes occurred in the incidence of ovarian cancer in women aged 50–70. Thus, the descriptive epidemiology of ovarian cancer in the United States is not supportive of a strong association between menopausal hormones and ovarian cancer.

More direct evidence comes from epidemiological studies concerning menopausal hormones and ovarian cancer[4–9]. One of the earliest studies suggested a two to threefold increase in risk, especially in women whose menopausal regimen included diethyl stilboestrol[4]. There then followed several studies suggesting that there was no association between menopausal hormones and ovarian cancer[5–7]. Weiss et al. reported an excess risk for ovarian cancer, especially of the endometrioid type, in women using menopausal hormones[8] and Cramer et al. suggested an association of borderline statistical significance in long-term users on unopposed cyclic regimens[9]. More specifically, the findings of the study by Cramer et al., which are shown in Table 3.1, indicated that women who had used menopausal hormones in cyclic fashion or for more than 5 years had exposed themselves to an approximately 2.5 times higher risk. In both of these instances the figures were of borderline statistical significance. Recently, there have been few studies and most of those which have been conducted relate to exposure in the era of unopposed oestrogen therapy. Overall, there does not appear to be any strong association between menopausal hormones and ovarian cancer; there may, at worst, be a weak association. Since the 1970s, newer regimens using combined oestrogen and progesterone therapy have been instituted and epidemiological studies to assess their impact on risk for ovarian cancer are now necessary. It is predicted, however, that these are likely to demonstrate a protective effect.

The basis for the prediction that combination menopausal therapy may be protective is drawn from studies on oral contraceptives and ovarian cancer. Numerous studies have now been conducted that demonstrate the protective effect of oral contraceptive use against ovarian cancer[10–15]. The most recent study by the Centers for Disease Control appears to indicate that there is a significantly decreased risk after as little as six months of use persisting for up to 15 years after use[15]. Several mechanisms have been proposed to account for the protective effect exerted by oral contraceptives. One suggestion is that oral contraceptives cause an interruption of ovulation and induce a

Table 3.1 RISK FOR OVARIAN CANCER ASSOCIATED WITH VARIOUS CATEGORIES OF MENOPAUSAL HORMONE USE[9]

Category of use	Cases (No.)	Controls (No.)	Adjusted RR*	95% confidence limits
Ever use				
None	145	153	1.0	–
Any	28	20	1.6	0.8, 2.9
Type				
Conjugated oestrogen	21	16	1.5	0.7, 2.9
Other	7	4	1.9	0.6, 6.2
Frequency				
Continuous	15	14	1.2	0.5, 2.5
Cyclic (or non-daily)	13	6	2.5	1.0, 6.4
Duration of use (years)				
≤ 1	9	6	1.5	0.5, 4.5
2–5	9	10	1.0	0.4, 2.5
> 5	9	4	2.8	0.9, 9.3

*Restricted to subjects over 40 and adjusted for parity.
RR = Relative Risk.

ovulatory rest, which is thought to be important in ovarian cancer aetiology[16]. A second possibility is that oral contraceptives may induce an increase in sex-hormone-binding globulins[17], while a third is that ovarian cancer may lower the levels of gonadotrophins[18]. In the remaining part of this discussion, evidence will be presented suggesting that this last mechanism is the most likely explanation for the protective effect of oral contraceptives and possibly of combination menopausal therapy.

Hypergonadotrophic hypogonadism a precursor of ovarian cancer?

It is our proposition that human ovarian cancer is largely a consequence of hypergonadotrophic hypogonadism. The main basis for this assertion lies in the parallels with animal models for inducing ovarian cancer. The majority of these animal models have been based on rodents and the primary model involved mechanisms that caused premature depletion of ovarian follicles, either through the use of radiation or polycyclic hydrocarbons, or as found in certain animal strains predisposed to a congenital deficiency of germ cells[19-21]. It was believed that such mechanisms were mediated via the high levels of gonadotrophins which followed depletion of follicles, since hypophysectomy prevented tumour development[22].

It has been argued that the animal models are irrelevant to human disease because the animal tumours were histologically different from human tumours. We contend that the stromal tumours in rodents are relevant to human epithelial tumours because there is much greater stromal-epithelial admixture in humans. This occurs as the human female ages and deep indentations of the surface epithelium dip into the surface of the ovary, eventually forming inclusion cysts. It is from these inclusion cysts that pathologists believe ovarian epithelial tumours arise[23]. A further reason why stromal tumours may be relevant to epithelial tumours is that stromal-epithelial interaction is probably involved in both differentiation and proliferation of many types of epithelium. Cunha summarized these data, noting that androgens induce differentiation of urogenital epithelium into either prostatic or vaginal epithelium depending upon the receptor status of the mesenchyme, and that oestradiol is not mitogenic for isolated mammary, uterine, or vaginal epithelial tissue grown in culture, but is mitogenic when the tissue is combined with homologous mesenchyme[24].

Hypergonadotrophic hypogonadism, epidemiological evidence in humans

It is instructive to examine whether there is any epidemiological evidence to support the relevance of the animal models to humans. As regards the role of radiation in the induction of human ovarian tumours, a large cohort study carried out in women irradiated for cervical cancer demonstrated a deficiency of ovarian tumours in the first 10 or 15 years following radiation treatment, but a significant excess beginning about 15 years after the radiation was received[25]. Women who survived the atomic bomb also showed a significant excess of ovarian tumours if they received the radiation dose when they were under 45 years of age and/or received a high dose close to the blast epicentre[26]. Thus, radiation may be associated with an increased risk for ovarian cancer if it is received at an early age when the ovaries are still functioning, if the dose is sufficient to induce the menopause, or if there has been a long latency period.

The second animal model for ovarian cancer tumorigenesis involves the use of certain chemicals, such as the polycyclic hydrocarbon dimethylbenzanthracene (DMBA), to cause premature depletion of ovarian follicles[20]. Humans may be exposed to such chemicals from tobacco smoke and there is at least one study that suggests an excess risk of ovarian tumours in smokers[27]. As in the case of radiation, the risk may be greater when the ovaries are exposed at an early age, such as might occur from smoking begun around the time of menarche or possibly from prenatal exposure to smoke from smoking parents.

Another model for ovarian cancer pathogenesis derives from several strains of mice born with a deficiency of germ cells and having high spontaneous rates of ovarian tumours[21]. This is a potentially important model for human ovarian tumorigenesis in that there is strong evidence that nulliparity is a risk factor for ovarian cancer and that a family history of ovarian cancer plays a significant role[9]. One hypothesis deserving of further study is that certain metabolic anomalies may predispose to risk for ovarian cancer. One basis for this hypothesis stems from the observation that hypergonadotrophic hypogonadism has been observed in patients with galactosaemia[28]. Thus, the study of enzymes related to galactose metabolism, including galactosetransferase, may provide evidence of one possible genetic mechanism for ovarian cancer and its link to infertility.

Another epidemiological observation consistent with the hypergonadotrophic hypogonadism model for ovarian cancer relates to mumps and ovarian cancer[29]. It has been found that ovarian cancer sufferers are significantly less likely to recall having had mumps parotitis, even though they have levels of mumps antibodies comparable to those in controls. This may mean that they have had a mumps infection that was not perceived as parotitis – in other words, mumps oophoritis. It is known that mumps is a cause of testicular failure, and menopause as a consequence of documented mumps oophoritis has also been described. Mumps may thus be another risk factor for ovarian cancer mediated via the ovarian failure pathway.

Finally, one of the strongest epidemiological associations for ovarian cancer is pregnancy history. Nulliparous patients are at greater risk for the disease than parous patients and the risk decreases as the number of children rises. Nulliparity may simply be a marker for underlying hypogonadism, but it is likely that pregnancy itself also plays a role. Pregnancy lowers gonadotrophins and it is possible that repeated pregnancies permanently alter the pituitary gland so as to change the secretion of trophic hormones in later life. The likely importance of gonadotrophin secretion in the peri-menopausal and post-menopausal period is suggested by a comparison of the age-specific incidence of ovarian cancer with the cumulative incidence of menopause. Stadel has commented on the striking graphic similarity between these, suggesting that ovarian cancer and the menopause are closely related[30].

Conclusion

If this paper has gone beyond the original brief to discuss the epidemiological evidence regarding menopausal hormones and ovarian cancer, the aim has been to place this issue in the broader perspective of underlying mechanisms. To conclude this discussion of ovarian cancer in relation to endogenous and exogenous hormones, some ideas are now advanced regarding the primary prevention of ovarian cancer.

First of all, we propose that the use of oral contraceptives, where medically appropriate in the 20s and 30s, would probably be beneficial in reducing ovarian cancer risk. Secondly, combination menopausal therapy, where medically appropriate, should be considered for administration to older women, especially those at risk for hypergonadotrophic hypogonadism. These may be nulliparous women, women who have never used oral contraceptives, or women with a family history of ovarian cancer. It is also likely that correction of the endocrine imbalances that occur during the peri-menopausal years may be more beneficial than post-menopausal therapy alone.

REFERENCES

1. Galli, M. C., Degiovanni, B. S., Nicoletti, G. et al. (1981). The occurrence of multiple steroid hormone receptors in disease-free and neoplastic human ovary. *Cancer*, **47**, 1297
2. Holt, J. A., Caputo, T. A., Kelly, K. M. et al. (1979). Estrogen and progestin binding in cytosol of ovarian carcinoma. *Obstet. Gynecol.*, **53**, 50
3. Gwinn, M. L., Lee, N. C. (1986). Trends in the incidence of endometrial and ovarian cancers. *MMWR*, **35**, 23SS–7SS

4. Hoover, R., Gray, L. A., Fraumeni, J. F. (1977). Stilbestrol and the risk of ovarian cancer. *Lancet*, **2**, 533
5. Annegers, J. F., Strom, H., Decker, D. G. et al. (1979). Ovarian cancer: incidence and case-control study. *Cancer*, **43**, 723
6. Hildreth, N. G., Kelsey, J. L., Livolsi, V. A. et al. (1981). An epidemiological study of epithelial carcinoma of the ovary. *Am. J. Epidemiol.*, **114**, 398
7. Francheschi, S., LaVecchia, C., Helmrich, S. P. et al. (1982). Risk factors for epithelial ovarian cancer in Italy. *Am. J. Epidemiol.*, **115**, 714
8. Weiss, N. S., Lyon, J. L., Krishnamurthy, S. et al. (1982). Noncontraceptive estrogen use and the occurrence of ovarian cancer. *J. Natl. Cancer Inst.*, **68**, 95
9. Cramer, D. W., Hutchison, G. K., Welch, W. R. et al. (1983). Determinants of ovarian cancer risk. I. Reproductive experiences and family history. *J. Natl. Cancer Inst.*, **71**, 711
10. Newhouse, M. L., Pearson, R. M., Fullerton, J. M. et al. (1977). A case/control study of carcinoma of the ovary. *Br. J. Prev. Soc. Med.*, **31**, 148
11. Willet, W. C., Bain, C., Hennekens, C. H. et al. (1981). Oral contraceptives and risk of ovarian cancer. *Cancer*, **48**, 1684
12. Weiss, N. S., Lyon, J. L., Liff, J. M. et al. (1981). Incidence of ovarian cancer in relation to the use of oral contraceptives. *Int. J. Cancer*, **28**, 669
13. Rosenberg, L., Shapiro, S., Slone, D. et al. (1982). Epithelial ovarian cancer and combination oral contraceptives. *J. Am. Med. Assoc.*, **247**, 3210
14. Cramer, D. W., Hutchison, G. B., Welch, W. R. et al. (1982). Factors affecting the association of oral contraceptives and ovarian cancer. *N. Engl. J. Med.*, **307**, 1047
15. The Cancer and Steroid Hormone Study. (1987). The reduction in risk of ovarian cancer associated with oral-contraceptive use. *N. Engl. J. Med.*, **316**, 650
16. Fathalla, M. F. (1971). Incessant ovulation – a factor in ovarian neoplasia? *Lancet*, **2**, 163
17. Pike, M. C., Chilvers, C. (1984). Hormonal contraception and breast cancer. In J. S. Scott, J. P. Wolf (Eds.). *Hormones and sexual factors in human cancer aetiology.* (Amsterdam: Elsevier Press)
18. Cramer, D. W., Welch, W. R. (1983). Determinants of ovarian cancer risk. II. Inferences regarding pathogenesis. *J. Natl. Cancer Inst.*, **71** (4), 717
19. Furth, J., Butterworth, J. S. (1936). Neoplastic diseases occurring among mice subjected to general irradiation with X-rays. *Am. J. Cancer*, **28**, 66
20. Jull, J. W., Streeter, D. J., Sutherland, L. (1966). The mechanism of induction of ovarian tumors in the mouse by 7.12-dimethyl-benz(a)athracene. I. Effect of steroid hormones and carcinogen concentration in vivo. *J. Natl. Cancer Inst.*, **37**, 409
21. Murphy, E. D., Russell, E. S. (1963). Ovarian tumorigenesis following

genic deletion of germ cells in hybrid mice. *Acta Unio Int. Cancer*, **19**, 779

22. Marchant, J. (1961). The effect of hypophysectomy on the development of ovarian tumours in mice treated with dimethylbenzanthracene. *Br. J. Cancer*, **15**, 821

23. Radisavljevic, S. V. (1977). The pathogenesis of ovarian inclusion cysts and cystomas. *Obstet. Gynecol.*, **49**, 424

24. Cunha, G. R., Bigsby, R. M., Cooke, P. S. et al. (1985). Stromal-epithelial interactions in adult organs. *Cell Differentiation*, **17**, 137

25. Day, N. E., Boice, J. D. (1983). Second cancer in relation to radiation treatment for cervical cancer. *IARC Publ.*, **52**, 163

26. Darby, S. C., Nakashima, E., Kato, H. (1985). A parallel analysis of cancer mortality among atomic bomb survivors and patients with ankylosing spondylitis given X-ray therapy. *J. Natl. Cancer Inst.*, **75**, 1

27. Doll, R., Gray, R., Hafner, B. et al. (1980). Mortality in relation to smoking: 22 years' observation on female British doctors. *Br. Med. J.*, **1**, 167

28. Kaufman, F. R., Kogut, M. D., Donnell, G. N. et al. (1981). Hypergonadotrophic hypogonadism in female patients with galactosemia. *N. Engl. J. Med.*, **304**, 994

29. Cramer, D. W., Welch, W. R., Cassells, S. (1983). Mumps, menarche, menopause and ovarian cancer. *Am. J. Obstet. Gynecol.*, **147**, 1

30. Stadel, B. V. (1975). The etiology and prevention of ovarian cancer. *Am. J. Obstet. Gynecol.*, **123**, 772

4

Advice to post-menopausal women

R. B. GREENBLATT AND A.-Z. TERAN

Introduction

In the ascent of man, the female of the species achieved the higher degree of perfection. If arrest of gonadal development occurs early in foetal life, a phenotypic female will result, regardless of the XY or XX chromosomal composition. Evidently the primary sex is female.

Woman is the stronger, not the weaker sex; it is she who endures pain better and shows greater resistance to infection and many debilitating diseases. Yet she alone, among all the species of the animal kingdom, experiences a menopause and the consequences of oestrogen deprivation.

The 'cessation of menses' in middle-aged women was alluded to by Pliny and other Roman writers as occurring at about 50 years of age, and this has not varied with time. The term 'menopause' was not introduced until the appearance of Gardanne's book in 1821, *De La Ménopause ou De L'Age Critique Des Femmes*[1]. Some five years earlier, he published "Avis aux femmes qui entrent dans l'âge critique" (Advice to women entering the critical age)[2]. Since then, much has changed. One thing is certain – the many myths and misconceptions that surround the menopause need to be addressed.

Clinicians abound who believe the menopause is a physiological event, a normal aging process, therefore oestrogen replacement therapy (ERT) is meddlesome and unnecessary. Presbyopia is a normal aging process, but none will deny the need for spectacles. To do nothing other than offer sympathy and assurance that the menopause will pass is tantamount to benign neglect. By such a strategem, the physician need not shoulder any guilt should a gynecic cancer or a cardiovascular accident intervene. My counsel to the post-menopausal woman is, "Avoid such a physician; seek out one who is knowledge-able about the hormone imbalance of the menopause". Today's women want to know why the menopause occurs, what it is and what it is not. How long does it last? Who should be treated? When, how, with what, and for how long? What are the advantages as well as the risks of oestrogen replacement therapy (ERT)?

The writer poses likely questions and attempts to answer them, realizing full well that the replies may be at variance with the opinions held by a few or even many of his peers. The answers are the crystal-lization of almost five decades of experience in the management of peri-menopausal woman.

What is the menopause?

When the ovarian follicles responsible for oestrogen production are exhausted or no longer functional, a train of symptoms are set in motion. The arrest of further menstruation is the critical happening that heralds a new era in a woman's progression through life. A more accurate term for this time of transition is the 'climacteric', since this includes the pre-menopausal and post-menopausal periods. It is a con-tinuum of events resulting from the oestrogen deficit. Thus, there is a pre-menopausal period that commences as the ovaries begin to falter, then the actual cessation of menses, followed by a post-menopausal period which ends at the time of demise. The climacteric is not a temporary event to be endured for only a few months or years. Many of the psychophysical and pathological aberrations, aided and abetted by the aging process, are due to oestrogen deprivation.

Can conception occur during the peri-menopause?

The climacteric celebrates a woman's passage from her reproductive years to freedom from the vicissitudes and hazards of childbearing. But is she entirely safe? A review of New York City statistics for 1940–50 revealed 20 births to women aged over 50 who presumed they were in the menopause[3]. In Great Britain, during 1981, there were 50 live births, 1 stillbirth and 15 abortions in women over 50 years of age[4]. Evidently a few residual follicles had been awakened and were still responsive. Perhaps the legend of biblical Sarah, who conceived after "It ceased to be with Sarah after the manner of women", may be more than apocryphal.

What does the hot flush signify?

Myths exist about the significance of the hot flush. One rampant belief is that once hot flushes disappear, the climacteric is over. Vasomotor symptoms appearing in the pre-menopausal period are often regarded as idiosyncratic and unrelated to the menopause. In fact, hot flushes may occur as a result of the relative lowering of oestrogen production, despite the regular or irregular bleeding periods which are often experienced for a few months or years before final cessation of menses. Some women never experience hot flushes, while others are plagued with them for from one to several decades.

The hypothalamus, having been sensitized by oestrogens over the years, shows its distemper when oestrogens are withdrawn. Increased levels of epinephrine and norepinephrine have been detected in the serum of women with severe hot flushes (Figure 4.1). The close association between vasomotor instability and hypothalamic dysfunction suggests that the metabolism of catecholamines and the level of oestrogen production are causally involved[5].

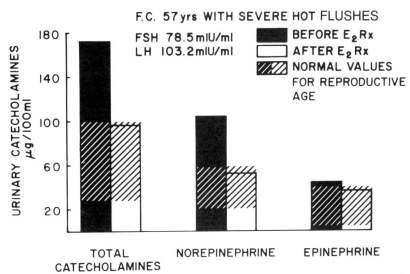

FIGURE 4.1 Urinary catecholamines increase during severe flushing and decrease after oestrogen therapy, suggesting a relationship between hypothalamic dysfunction and hormones.

What are the manifestations of the menopause?

The current consensus is that only vasomotor instability (hot flushes, night sweats) and atrophic vaginitis are true manifestations of the menopause – all other symptoms are commentary. For a long time such metabolic disorders as osteoporosis, lipidaemia and skin collagen loss were not considered part of the menopausal picture and nor were neurogenic disturbances – depression, anxiety, migrainoid headaches and insomnia[6]. Certainly, incontinence and nocturia unaccounted for by anatomical changes or bacterial infection were not even remotely regarded as being associated with hormonal imbalance[7]. However, the presence of oestrogen receptors in the lower urinary tract has been reported[8]. The epithelial cells lining the urethra and anterior third of the bladder undergo similar atrophic changes during the menopause to those of the vagina (Figure 4.2).

For a long time 'purists' have ridiculed the concept that many of the psychosomatic disturbances observed during the menopause are hormone-related. Dopamine and norepinephrine play a significant role in modulating mood, behaviour, and hypothalamic-pituitary function. Monoamine oxidase (MAO) concentrations reach prodigious levels in depressed menopausal women[9]. Concentrations of dopamine in the hypothalamus decrease and those of norepinephrine increase following castration[10]. Moreover, the levels of tryptophan – a precursor of serotonin – are low in the serum of depressed menopausal women and the rise following oestrogen therapy parallels clinical improvement (Table 4.1)[11,12]. Large doses of oestrogens (5–25 mg of conjugated oestrogens) lower MAO concentrations, with corresponding improvements in Hamilton Scale scores[13]. Because women on ERT often sleep better, it was alleged that this was due to improvement in vasomotor instability[14]. It has been shown, however, that the ratio of norepinephrine to serotonin is associated with rapid eye movement (REM) sleep patterns[15]. As to non-bacterial urinary disorders, the writer tried many years ago to reduce the size of massive uterine fibromyomata with androgens; he failed but found that the incidental nocturia was alleviated. Androgens as well as oestrogens may ameliorate urinary symptoms in many menopausal women[16].

When, how and what hormones should be prescribed?

Conventional thinking is that if a woman is placed on ERT, the treatment should be for the minimum period of time, varying from

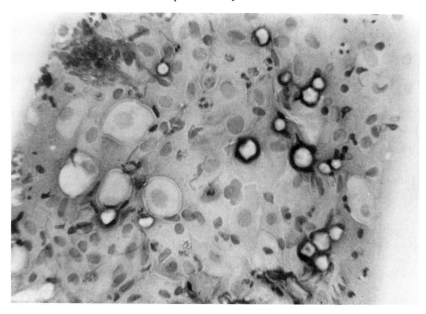

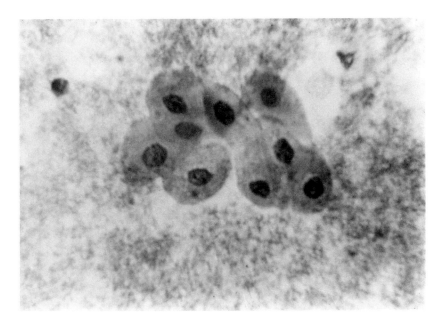

FIGURE 4.2 Smears made from the sediment of a urine sample and from the vagina of a menopausal woman reveal similar parabasal cells resulting from oestrogen deficiency.

Table 4.1 SERUM TRYPTOPHAN VALUES IN MENOPAUSAL WOMEN ON OES-
TROGEN THERAPY**

	Free (4.2–6.0 Umol/ml)		Total (34.3–48.3 Umol/ml)	
	Before	After	Before	After
Depressed	3.78	4.78*	35.33	41.33
	±0.02	±0.37	±0.67	±5.93
	$n = 160$	$n = 104$	$n = 160$	$n = 104$
Non-depressed	5.12	5.79	44.80	45.10
	±0.34	±0.87	±5.93	±3.01
	$n = 20$	$n = 20$	$n = 20$	$n = 20$

Free and total tryptophan levels are much lower in depressed than in non-depressed
women. Following administration of oestrogens the rise in serum tryptophan parallels the
improvement in the depressive state.

only months to one or two years at most and that the oestrogen should
be administered orally, at minimum doses and in cyclic fashion (21–25
days per month). Such advice is not always practical – some women
require continuous therapy, either because symptoms return during the
treatment-free period or they develop oestrogen-withdrawal headaches[17]. Others need larger doses and some require ERT for years,
feeling 'let down' without it. Furthermore, ERT is not necessarily
directed at assuaging hot flushes and night sweats alone, it may also be
aimed at allaying emotional instability and lessening the metabolic
insult produced by chronic hypo-oestrogenism. Moreover, if a woman
does not tolerate or respond satisfactorily to oral therapy, the use of
parenteral therapy is in order, i.e. injections, pellet implants, vaginal
creams, suppositories, or dermal patches, for as long as the patient's
well-being calls for such support.

Do progestogens protect against endometrial cancer?

When oestrogens are employed, it is prudent to offer cyclic courses of
an oral progestogen to induce orderly withdrawal bleeding and protect
the patient from increased risk of endometrial cancer[18]. Unfortunately,
about 15% of women suffer premenstrual syndrome-like symptoms
during progestogen therapy and consequently refuse to take it[19,20].

Accordingly, the suggestion has been made that only 5 mg of medroxy-progesterone acetate (the usual dose is 10 mg) should be administered every third month for 10 days to induce shedding of the endo-metrium[21]. It has been my practice, where there is a progestogen idiosyncracy, to change the preparation, reduce the course to 5–7 days, and if necessary cut the dosage by half. If any spotting or abnormal bleeding should intervene, an endometrial biopsy (office procedure) is immediately performed to rule out atypical hyperplasia or endometrial cancer.

How should oestrogens be prescribed for women with an intact uterus?

There is a growing consensus that progestogens are not a necessary adjunct to ERT. The risk of endometrial cancer, though real, has been exaggerated; the risk is actually small (5 ± 3-fold), so that 955 ± 3 women per thousand on oestrogen therapy do not develop cancer. Furthermore, the endometrial cancer that develops in women while on oestrogens is usually of the mature type; it is detected early because of abnormal bleeding, and the prognosis following hysterectomy is excellent[22]. An analysis of the staging of the cancers reported by Smith et al. in 1975 revealed a dramatic difference in favour of the oestrogen-treated women (Table 4.2)[23]. Endometrial cancers in non-oestrogen treated women are more frequently invasive and the prognosis much poorer.

Admittedly, the evidence is strong that progestogens prevent hyperplasia and decrease the incidence of endometrial cancer[24–27]. Endometrial cancers do nevertheless occur. Perfect protection has not yet been achieved.

In the past few years, small continuous doses of an oestrogen-progestogen regimen have been suggested with a view to inducing endometrial atrophy and permanent amenorrhoea. Unfortunately, breakthrough spotting and bleeding occurs during the first four months in about 40% of cases, although by the end of a year only 10% continue to experience breakthrough bleeding. This is an area that requires much more exploration[28,29].

When women are adamant about not reviving menstrual periods, they should be accommodated by prescribing 0.3–0.625 mg of conjugated oestrogens or the equivalent from Monday to Friday of each

Table 4.2 HISTOLOGY OF ENDOMETRIAL PATHOLOGY IN CASES OF SMITH ET AL (1975)*

Stage	Oestrogen Group	Non-Oestrogen Group
0	16	7
1	129	115
2	6	20
3	2	15
4	0	7
Total	153	164

*From Studd (1976) with kind permission of the author and the editor of the *British Medical Journal*.

Smith et al.,[23] who warned of the association of oestrogens and endometrial cancer, provided the staging of endometrial cancers in their oestrogen and non-oestrogen treated controls. Note that invasive cancer (stages 3 and 4) is much more frequent in the controls than in those receiving oestrogen replacement therapy.

week. Often, 1.25–2.5 mg of methyltestosterone is added to the regimen. The combination is well tolerated and arrhenomimetic phenomena are rare.

Does adequate calcium intake prevent osteoporosis?

The public has been taken in by the media blitz claiming that a high calcium intake will prevent bone loss. To some extent the commercial advertisements are a deceit, if not actually fraudulent. Calcium retards bone resorption but does not prevent osteoporosis. Oestrogen is the cement that binds the building blocks (calcium) together. Non-oestrogen users have a 2 to 3-fold fracture risk (hip, radius)[30]. Cyclic oestrogen and progestogen therapy started before the third post-menopausal year not only prevents bone loss but actually increases bone density[31,32]. With the abrupt cessation of hormone therapy, regressive bone change sets in rapidly[33]. In the osteoporotic, ERT should be continued forever. Once marked osteoporosis has set in, oestrogen and progestogen administration may prevent further bone decay, but does not appear to be able to restore bone mass (Figure 4.3). Preventive steps comprise oestrogens, calcium and exercise.

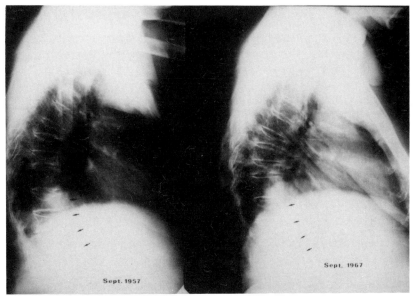

FIGURE 4.3
(a) Severe osteoporosis in a 49-year-old woman with primary amenorrhoea.
(b) Ten years of oestrogen-progestogen therapy prevented a further deterioration.
After thirty years of continuous hormonal therapy no new compression fractures or further bone decay had occurred.

Do oestrogens lessen the risk of cardiovascular disease?

The Framington group claims that the risk of myocardial infarction (MI), cerebral accidents, phlebitis and hypertension increases in women on ERT[34]. Others are in favour of ERT as a means of reducing the incidence of cardiovascular disease[35]. The final verdict is not yet in[36].

The mechanism by which oestrogens are alleged to exert their protective action is thought to be mediated through reversal of low-density to high-density lipoprotein (LDL : HDL) ratios. Oestrogens favourably restore this ratio in nonsmoking menopausal women to the value seen during their reproductive years. While oestrogens are beneficial, certain progestogens (norethindrone, norgestrel) have deleterious effects, but pure progesterone – in the form of injectables, suppositories and oral (micronized) tablets – does not. However, Shargil found that low-dose oral contraceptives (triphasic) did not interfere with lipoprotein patterns in peri-menopausal women after three years' use[37].

Is sexual dysfunction a psychosexual problem?

The belief is generally current that depression, anxiety and the empty-nest syndrome are at the core of sexual dysfunction in the menopausal woman. It has been suggested that psychiatric help and counselling, rather than hormonal therapy, should be tried to remedy the problem. Admittedly, psychogenic factors are paramount, but ERT frequently lessens depression and anxiety and restores libidinous drives (Table 4.3). Furthermore, dyspareunia due to dryness and atrophy of the vaginal mucosa may be greatly reduced by oestrogens. When ERT fails, androgens in non-virilizing doses, with or without oestrogens, may provide surprising results – increasing well-being, energy level and sexual fantasies[38,39].

Androgens in physiological doses are not anti-oestrogenic or causes of pharmacological mayhem as claimed[40] – they act synergistically[41]. Hormone assays of peripheral and ovarian vein blood reveal that androgen production is involved in the body economy (Table 4.4). Testosterone has been implicated as a cause of increases in LDL concentrations. This is only a half-truth. While it is indeed so for substantial doses (5–10+ mg/day) of synthetic oral androgens (methyl-

Table 4.3 LIBIDO RESPONSE IN DEPRESSED MENOPAUSAL PATIENTS ON ESTROGEN THERAPY*

	Excellent	Moderate	Non-Responsive
Depression n=160	66 (41.25%)	69 (43.13%)	25 (15.63%)
Libido n=112	39 (34.82%)	52 (46.43%)	21 (18.75%)

*2 Estradiol pellets (25 mg. each)

Oestrogens lessen depression, with subsequent return of libido. In non-depressed patients, adjunctive androgen therapy is usually necessary.

testosterone, etc.), it is not the case when pure testosterone (pellets or injectables) are employed[42,43]. Small doses of synthetic oral androgens (1.25–2.5 mg) have been prescribed together with 0.3–0.625 mg of conjugated oestrogens or oestrone sulphate preparations without causing significant changes in lipid fractions.

Table 4.4

MEAN ± VALUES OF PERIPHERAL AND OVARIAN VEIN ESTRADIOL (E_2), Δ^4-ANDROSTENEDIONE (Δ^4A) AND TESTOSTERONE (T) LEVELS IN 11 MENOPAUSAL AND 10 NORMAL WOMEN

	Peripheral			Ovarian		
	E_2 (pg/ml)	Δ^4A (ng/ml)	T (ng/ml)	E_2 (pg/ml)	Δ^4A (ng/ml)	T (ng/ml)
Normal	41 ± 15 *					
	58 ± 11 * *	1.47	0.28 ± 0.4	83.1	1.72	0.87
Menopausal	21.26 ± 2.18	1.09 ± 0.10	0.53 ± 0.06	30.52 ± 2.49	2.2 ± 0.17	0.91 ± 0.13

* Follicular phase
* * Luteal phase

Serum hormone levels (peripheral and ovarian) suggest that androgens probably play an important role in a woman's physiology. Note that ovarian △-4-androsterone and testosterone levels are higher in post-menopausal than in normal women.

Conclusions

The questions a woman may ask should be answered frankly but not dogmatically. She should be made aware that hormones will not prevent aging, but may slow the aging process; they will not erase the wrinkled brow, raise the sagging breast, or straighten the hunching back. Hormones are psychotonic agents which may moderate emotional swings and temper the racing mind. While it may be difficult to prove that the many psychosomatic aberrations of the menopause are hormone-dependent, they are frequently hormone-responsive[44]. The imbalance of the autonomic nervous system, the neurogenic disturbances and the metabolic disorders continue in mild to severe form to the end of life. Although the hormonal environment can be improved, many women are still unable to cope and to adjust. They envision goals which remain forever inaccessible; they recall bygone charms ('charmes perdus') and the mystique of full-fashioned womanhood they once possessed. The life history and destiny of every woman are dependent to a great degree on the intensity and duration of her ovarian activity.

The advantages of hormone replacement therapy far outweigh the risks. The prescribing of oestrogens, a balanced diet, and exercise, is good preventive medicine. Régine Sitruk-Ware captures the essence of the problem in her up-to-date book, *La Ménopause*, when she states that although the arrest of ovarian function is an inevitable 'physiological' event, the consequences of the oestrogen decline become pathological and justify a preventive approach[45]. Indeed, hormone replacement therapy may delay the inevitable, refresh the spirit, contribute to the enjoyment of life and bring nearer to fruition Margaret Mead's pronouncement: "The most creative force in the world is the menopausal woman with zest".

REFERENCES

1. de Gardanne, C. P. L. (1821). *De La Ménopause ou De L'Age Critique Des Femmes*. (Paris: Méquignon-Marvis)
2. de Gardanne, C. P. L. (1816). *Avis Aux Femmes Qui Entrent Dans L'Age Critique*. (Paris, Gabon)
3. Kaufman, S. A. (1969). Fertility and conception after age forty. *Obstet. Gynecol., N.Y.*, **3**, 288
4. Guillebaud, J. (1985). Contraception for older women. *J. Obstet. Gynecol.*, **5** (Suppl. 2), S70
5. Casper, R. F., Yen, S. S. C. (1981). Menopausal flushes: effect of pituitary gonadotrophin desensitization by a potent luteinizing hormone-releasing factor agonist. *J. Clin. Endocrinol. Metab.*, **53**, 1056
6. Brincat, M., Moniz, C. F., Studd, J. W. W. et al. (1985). The long term effects of the menopause and of administration of sex hormones on skin collagen and skin thickness. *Br. J. Obstet. Gynaecol.*, **92**, 256
7. Smith, P. J. B. (1976). The effect of estrogens on bladder function in the female. In Campbell, S. (ed.). *The Management of the Menopause and Post-Menopausal Years*, p. 291. (Lancaster: MTP Press)
8. Josif, C. S., Batra, S., Elk, A. et al. (1981). Estrogen receptors in the human female lower urinary tract. *Am. J. Obstet. Gynecol.*, **141**, 817
9. Yen, S. S. C. (1977). The biology of the menopause. *J. Reprod. Med.*, **18**, 287

10. Donoso, A. L., Stephano, I. J. E., Biscardi, A. M. et al. (1967). Effects of castration on hypothalamic catecholamines. *Am. J. Physiol.*, **212**, 737

11. Aylward, M. (1975). Estrogens, plasma tryptophan levels in perimenopausal patients. In Campbell, S. (ed.). *The Management of the Menopause and Post Menopausal Years*, p. 137. (London: University Park Press)

12. Greenblatt, R. B., Chaddha, J. S., Teran, A.-Z. et al. (1985). Aphrodisiacs. In Iversen, S. D. (ed.). *Psychopharmacology: Recent Advances and Future Prospects*, p. 289. (Oxford: Oxford University Press)

13. Klaiber, E. L., Broverman, D. M., Vogel, W. et al. (1972). Effects of estrogen therapy on MAO activity and EEG during responses in depressed women. *Am. J. Psychiatr.*, **28**, 1492

14. Campbell, S., Whitehead, M. (1977). Oestrogen therapy in the menopausal syndrome. In Greenblatt, R. B., Studd, J. W. W. (eds.). *Clinics in Obstetrics and Gynaecology.* (London: W. B. Saunders)

15. Webb, W. B. (1969). Partial and differential sleep deprivation. In Kayes, A. (ed.). *Sleep physiology and pathology*, p. 221. (Philadelphia: Lippincott)

16. Greenblatt, R. B. (1943). Influence of pellets of testosterone propionate on nocturia. *J. Am. Med. Assoc.*, **121**, 17

17. Dennerstein, L., Burrows, G. D., Hyman, G. J. et al. (1979). Hormone therapy and affect. *Maturitas*, **1**, 247

18. Gambrell, R. D. (1982). Clinical use of progestins in the menopausal patient. *J. Reprod. Med.*, **27**, 531

19. Magos, A. L., Collins, W. P., Studd, J. W. W. (1984). Management of the premenstrual syndrome by subcutaneous implants of oestradiol. *J. Psychosom. Obstet. Gynecol.*, **3**, 93

20. Greenblatt, R. B., Teran, A.-Z., Barfield, W. E. et al. (1987). Premenstrual syndrome. *Stress Med.* (In Press)

21. Haspels, A. (1984). Abstract – *4th International Congress on the Menopause*, Orlando, Florida, USA

22. MacDonald, P. C. (1986). Editorial, Estrogen plus progestin in postmenopausal women – *Act. II. N. Engl. J. Med.* **315**, 959

23. Smith, D. C., Prentice, R., Thompson, D. J. et al. (1975). Association of exogenous estrogen and endometrial carcinoma. *N. Engl. J. Med.*, **293**, 1164

24. Gambrell, R. D. Jr. (1977). Estrogens, progestogens and endometrial cancer. *J. Reprod. Med.*, **18**, 301

25. Whitehead, M. I. (1978). The effect of oestrogens and progesterone on the postmenopausal endometrium. *Maturitas*, **1**, 87

26. Thom, M. H., White, P. J., Williams, R. N. et al. (1976). Prevention and treatment of endometrial oestrogens and endometrial cancer. In Beard, R. J. (ed.). *The Menopause.* (Lancaster: MTP Press)

27. Greenblatt, R. B., Gambrell, R. D. Jr., Stoddard, L. D. (1982). The protective role of progesterone in the prevention of endometrial cancer. *Path. Res. Pract.*, **174**, 297

28. Magos, A. L., Brincat, M., Studd, J. W. W. et al. (1985). Amenorrhea and endometrial atrophy with continuous oral estrogen and progestogen therapy in postmenopausal women. *Obstet. Gynecol.*, **65**, 496

29. Staland, B. (1981). Continuous treatment with natural oestrogens and progestogens. A method to avoid endometrial stimulation. *Maturitas*, **3**, 145

30. Horsman, A., Gallagher, J. C., Simpson, M. et al. (1977). Prospective trial of estrogen and calcium in postmenopausal women. *Br. Med. J.*, **2**, 798

31. Christiansen, C., Christensen, M. S., MacNair, P. et al. (1980). Prevention of early postmenopausal bone loss. *Eur. J. Clin. Invest.*, **10**, 273

32. Nachtigall, L. E., Nachtigall, R. H., Nachtigall, R. D. et al. (1979). Estrogen replacement therapy: I. A ten year prospective study on the relationship to osteoporosis. *Obstet. Gynecol.*, **53**, 277

33. Lindsay, R., Hart, D. M., MacLean, A. et al. (1978). Bone response to termination of estrogen treatment. *Lancet*, **1**, 1325

34. Gordon, T., Kannel, W. B., Hjortland, M. C. et al. (1978). Menopause and coronary heart disease. The Framington Study. *Am. Int. Med.*, **89**, 157

35. Ross, R. K., Paganini-Hill, A., Mack, T. M. et al. (1981). Menopausal estrogen therapy and protection from ischemic heart disease. *Lancet*, **1**, 858

36. Schiff, I., Ryan, K. J. (1980). Benefits of estrogen replacement therapy. *Obstet. Gynecol. Survey,* Williams and Wilkins

37. Shargil, A. A. (1986). Hormone replacement therapy in perimenopausal women with a triphasic contraceptive compound – A three year prospective study. *Int. J. Fertil.*, **30**, 11

38. Sherwin, B. B., Gelfand, M. M. (1985). Differential symptom response to parenteral estrogen and/or androgen administration in the surgical menopause. *Am. J. Obstet. Gynecol.*, **151**, 152

39. Studd, J. W. W., Collins, W. P. (1977). Oestradiol and testosterone implants in the treatment of psychosexual problems in the post-menopausal woman. *Br. J. Gynaecol.*, **84**, 314

40. Hamblen, E. C. (1941). Rationale for androgenic therapy in gynecology. *J. Clin. Endocrinol.*, **1**, 180

41. a Greenblatt, R. B. (1942). Androgenic therapy in women. Letter to the Editor. *J. Clin. Endocrinol.*, **2**, 655
    b Greenblatt, R. B. (1942). Hormone factors in libido. *J. Clin. Endocrinol.*, **3**, 305

42. Teran, A.-Z., Greenblatt, R. B., Chaddha, J. S. (1987). Changes in lipoproteins with various sex steroids. *Obstet. Gynecol. Clin. N. Amer.*, **14**, 107

43. Sherwin, B. B., Gelfand, M. M., Schucher, R. et al. (1987). Postmenopausal estrogen and androgen replacement and lipoprotein lipid concentrations. *Am. J. Obstet. Gynecol.*, **147**, 414

44. Lauritzen, C. (1973). The management of the pre-menopausal and the

post-menopausal patient. In van Keep, P. A., Lauritzen, C. (eds.). *Frontiers of Hormone Res., Vol 2., Aging and Estrogens,* p. 2. (Basel: Karger)

45. Sitruk-Ware, R. (1986). *La Ménopause.* (Paris: Flammarion Médecine)

5

Cost-effectiveness of hormonal replacement therapy

B. G. WREN

The cost of caring for post-menopausal women is becoming an intolerable burden for the taxpaying community, and unless efforts are made to restrict the number of medical consultations entailed demands will soon be made for older women to be treated differently to their affluent younger sisters. At present, women over the age of 60 years (7.8% of the Australian population) account for over 25% of the total health-care expenditure and occupy 40% of all available health-care beds. This disproportionate use of facilities by older women occurs for a number of reasons:

(a) Women live longer than men. There is a difference of about 7 years in the average age of death in favour of women, which means that the very elderly age groups comprise a larger number of females than males.

(b) Women tend to suffer from osteoporosis and bone fractures more frequently than men. This is believed to be partly the result of calcium loss caused by post-menopausal oestrogen deficiency. Fractures of the hip, wrist and spine are respectively three, four and ten times more common in females than in males.

(c) Women undergoing the menopause suffer from a number of debilitating problems, including hot flushes, insomnia, tiredness, irritability, panic, agitation, feelings of despondency, depression and inability to cope. These symptoms take them to their doctor for repeated medical consultations where they are often given inappropriate and expensive medication to relieve these 'symptoms'.

(d) After the menopause there is an increasing rate of cardiac disease among women and the graph of the incidence of myocardial infarction in Australian women exactly parallels that of males, except that it is 10 years later. This delay in the onset of myocardial infarction is thought to be due to the protective influence of oestrogen on the total cholesterol: high-density lipoprotein (HDL) cholesterol ratio.

(e) Women tend to marry men who are 4.2 years older than themselves and because men die some 7 years earlier than females it is often found that women live their last 10 years in a lonely and depressed situation. They take up beds and services but gain little enjoyment from life. They are often sedated, may have incapacitating fractures, suffer incontinence, or have debilitating bed sores, pneumonia or urinary infections. Their senescence is neither graceful nor dignified. They feel depressed, frustrated and angry, but few in the community care. Nevertheless, the cost of the health care they require is enormous. In Australia the total cost of the health care provided for some 600,000 women over 65 years of age exceeds a quarter of the total health-care budget. Unless positive action is taken soon the country will no longer be able to afford its older citizens. The best chance of reducing these health-care costs clearly lies in prophylactic medicine.

Prophylaxis of the diseases of aging women

One of the most significant means of reducing the rising tide of health-care costs for the elderly could be voluntary, long-term hormonal replacement therapy. However, before deciding that this should be recommended for all post-menopausal women, it is important to examine the cost-effectiveness of such treatment. This involves two sets of considerations – firstly, the cost of a therapy regimen versus the savings to be gained from the prophylaxis of disease and, secondly, the risk of inducing adverse side effects versus the physical, mental and sexual well-being to be gained from hormonal replacement therapy.

Therapy regimen

Most workers in the field of hormonal replacement therapy are now agreed that a naturally metabolized oestrogen with a non-androgenic progestogen given in a cyclic or continuous manner is the ideal regimen for post-menopausal therapy. In this context Premarin, Progynova and Ogen are the three most frequently used oral preparations, while micronized oestradiol, administered either orally, transdermally or vaginally, is also becoming popular. The progestogens of choice are those which exert an adequate protective effect on the endometrium and breasts without producing abnormal changes in blood lipid or blood pressure readings.

For the purposes of this paper Progynova and Provera respectively have been taken as representative examples of the oestrogens and progestogens commonly used to treat post-menopausal problems.

If every one of the 2,030,000 post-menopausal women in Australia were treated with Progynova for 21 days in each 28-day cycle, with 5 mg Provera added from day 10 to day 21, the cost would amount to $72,000,000 annually.

Add to this sum the charges for two medical consultations each year ($121,800,000) and the total annual cost involved in administering therapy rises to about $194,000,000. In addition, it is estimated that approximately 3–5% of patients under therapy each year will experience abnormal bleeding necessitating diagnostic curettage. Since more than 35% of Australian women will have had a hysterectomy by the age of 60 years, it is likely that about 60,000 women will require a curettage each year. The medical fees for a curettage are around $165.00 (surgeon plus anaesthetist), while inpatient fees are about $125.00. The total annual cost of performing curettages for these 60,000 women would thus not exceed $20,000,000.

Accordingly, the overall financial cost of administering hormonal replacement therapy to every post-menopausal woman in Australia would amount to about $215,000,000 each year.

The potential savings to be achieved by such a scheme can be measured by calculating the cost of the reduced incidence of cancer of the endometrium, the reduced risk of osteoporosis and the reduced frequency of attendance for medical consultation. There might also be a marked reduction in the risk of developing myocardial infarction and this will also be discussed together with the estimated figures involved.

Carcinoma of the endometrium

Based on information from the New South Wales Cancer Registry it would appear that the risk of developing cancer of the uterus in Australia is about 1 : 1200 after the menopause. Oestrogen alone may increase this risk to about 1 : 200, but when it is combined with an appropriate progestogen for 12 or more days each cycle the risk is reduced to less than 1 : 2000.

Thus, the treatment of post-menopausal women with an appropriate hormonal replacement regimen should reduce the number of uterine cancers by some 500–600 annually. The cost savings resulting from not having to treat 500 cancers of the uterus would be about $5,000,000 annually.

Osteoporosis

When a fracture of the hip occurs in Australia the following sequence of events takes place for both male and female patients:

(a) They are admitted to hospital, where appropriate initial steps are taken to make the diagnosis, including X-rays and other investigations.

(b) The hip is 'pinned' under general anaesthetic.

(c) The patient then spends 29.7 days in hospital, receiving initial post-operative care and convalescence.

(d) About 20–25% are returned to their own homes where active therapy is carried out to achieve recovery of function – usually over about 12 weeks. Very few of these people die.

(e) About 70–80% are transferred to nursing or convalescent homes, ostensibly to receive the same active therapy and support.

(f) Of those transferred to nursing or convalescent homes about one-third die within 12 months without ever regaining mobility.

(g) Of those who do regain mobility in nursing and convalescent homes, only about half ever actually leave the home (about 25% of the total in the case of hip fractures).

Of all those who enter hospital with a fractured hip, about one-third die within 12 months after considerable expenditure, while only about 40% regain adequate mobility. The remaining quarter of the patients continue to be a heavy financial burden on the community until they too die from some intercurrent illness a year or more after their initial fracture.

The cost of osteoporosis

Inpatient care for a hip fracture victim has been calculated to cost approximately $345.00 daily for 29.7 days (or $10,250). Convalescent care in a nursing home for an average period of 12 weeks costs $3,500, and rehabilitation and social work accounts for a further $750.00. The first 16 weeks of care following a fracture of the hip therefore costs about $14,500.

However, since almost 50% of all patients remain in a nursing home and require intensive medical, nursing and physiotherapeutic care at a further cost of about $8,500 each, the total individual average annual cost for fracture of the hip is about $20,000. As there are approximately 14,500 hip fractures each year, this injury alone costs $290,000,000. Add to this the cost of the management of wrist, spine, pelvic and other long bone fractures associated with osteoporosis and it is easy to conclude that health-care costs for osteoporosis alone would exceed $400,000,000 annually.

If all associated medical problems, such as respiratory difficulties, gastrointestinal compression, urinary infections and bed sores are also considered, the annual cost of caring for osteoporotic fractures escalates considerably, towards half a billion dollars annually. Any means of reducing this cost accordingly warrants careful consideration.

Reduction of osteoporosis costs through hormonal replacement therapy

In 1984, Australia had a population of approximately 15,500,000 and of these about 2,030,000 were females over the age of 50 years. Of some 10,800 women who fractured a hip in that year, most (91%) were over the age of 65 years. During the same period only 2,250 men of the same age suffered a similar problem. If an appropriate therapy regimen including hormonal replacement therapy had been instituted from the time of the menopause it is estimated that the rate of fracture of the hip among women would have been at least as low as that for men. On the basis of the male fracture rate it is calculated that such a regimen would have prevented at least 5,640 hip fractures, as well as some 10,000 wrist and at least 50,000 spinal crush fractures. The savings in health-care costs would thus have exceeded $250,000,000 over the year.

Myocardial infarction

Data obtained from the Bureau of Census and Statistics and from the National Heart Foundation indicate that there were about 12,800 female deaths due to coronary heart disease in 1984. A large number of these were related to atherosclerotic changes in the coronary vessels. It is thought that for every death from myocardial infarction there are at least four other non-fatal cases, from which it is estimated that about 60,000 women suffered a heart attack in Australia in 1984.

Cost of atherosclerosis

Of the 60,000 victims of the 'heart attacks' that occur in women each year, about 12,000 die within two weeks of admission to hospital, while the average hospital stay of the remainder is 17.3 days.

The average cost of inpatient care for myocardial infarction in Australia is $350.00 daily, so the total annual cost for treating women with ischaemic heart disease is about $360,000,000. A number of researchers have suggested that oestrogen may have a prophylactic role to play in reducing the risk of atherosclerosis and both Stampfer[1] and Henderson[2] have produced evidence to suggest that oestrogen reduces the rate of infarction by about one-half to two-thirds. Accordingly, if all Australian women received hormonal replacement therapy from the menopause onwards, the potential cost saving would be in the vicinity of $200,000,000 annually.

Cost-effectiveness

Based on the assumptions made, it appears that the cost of administering hormonal replacement therapy to over 2,000,000 women would be about $215,000,000 annually. This calculation takes into account the cost of oestrogen and progestogen ($72,000,000), two medical consultations each year ($121,800,000) and surgical intervention in a small number of cases ($20,000,000).

The savings would include a reduction in the incidence of cancer of the uterus ($5,000,000), a lower incidence of osteoporosis fractures ($250,000,000) and a potential reduction in ischaemic heart disease ($200,000,000).

Other potential savings which cannot be easily evaluated are a possible reduction in the number of medical consultations and a marked reduction in the use of psychotrophic and other medication prescribed for distressed older women. Indeed, Hammond[3] has reported a halving of the need for medical consultation and a similar reduction in prescription requirements for post-menopausal women receiving hormonal replacement therapy.

Cost-benefits

In discussing the cost-benefits to women, the main consideration is the improvement in the quality of life versus the risk of inducing an abnormality.

Women undergoing the menopause who suffer from hot flushes, sweats, palpitations, insomnia, tiredness, irritability, confusion, depression, panic, loss of libido, a sore dry vagina or a general feeling of despair will desperately seek a cure for their problems. Oestrogen has long been known to relieve the symptoms, but when given alone it was found to increase the risk of cancer of the uterus and was also associated with abnormal bleeding patterns. The risk to women was considered unacceptably high.

More recently, the significant role of progestogens has been highlighted. The use of cyclic or continuous low-dose natural oestrogens with continuous or cyclic non-androgenic progestogens has now led to a marked reduction in the risk of endometrial cancer and probably also of breast cancer. More significantly, it has brought about a reduction in the incidence of osteoporosis and probably atherosclerosis. The use of continuous non-androgenic progestogens with cyclic or continuous oestrogens results in minimal or no withdrawal bleeding and almost certainly eliminates the risk of uterine cancer.

When the benefit of the improved quality of life is added to the reduced risk of cancer, osteoporosis and ischaemic heart disease, the scales weigh heavily in favour of advising women to take hormonal replacement therapy from the time of the menopause.

The cost-effectiveness of the therapy also militates strongly in favour of treatment and every government should therefore seriously consider the enormous potential savings in health-care costs to be achieved from promoting prophylactic hormonal replacement therapy.

REFERENCES

1. Stampfer, M. J., Willett, W. C., Colditz, C. et al. (1985). A prospective study of post menopausal estrogen therapy and coronary heart disease. *N.*

Engl. J. Med., **313**, 1044

2. Henderson, B. E. (1984). Estrogen Replacement Therapy and the risk of arteriosclerotic cardiovascular disease. *Proceedings from a Symposium on Estrogen Replacement Therapy*. Abbott Laboratories Open Round Table Conference, San Francisco

3. Hammond, C. B., Jelovsek, F. R., Lee, K. L. et al. (1979). Effects of long-term estrogen replacement therapy I. – Metabolic Effects. *Am. J. Obstet. Gyn.*, **133**, 525

6

Consequences and treatment of early loss of ovarian function

M. I. WHITEHEAD AND M. CUST

Introduction

Generally speaking, medical reviews can be classified into (1) those which are comprehensive and consider all aspects of a particular topic, and (2) those which concentrate on specific areas of a topic. The latter often appear in response to newly acquired information becoming a major public health issue, as testified by the numerous reviews produced in the late 1970s on the association between unopposed oestrogen use and endometrial cancer in postmenopausal women.

Ten years ago it might have been possible to produce, in one book chapter, a comprehensive review on the incidence, aetiology, consequences and treatment of premature gonadal failure and premature menopause. However, the recent expansion in knowledge now precludes this; indeed, one entire supplement of *Seminars in Reproductive Endocrinology*[1], over 100 pages, was recently devoted exclusively to premature gonadal failure. This present review, therefore, is selective and will concentrate on the consequences of the oestrogen deficiency which follows ovarian failure, and on the establishment of pregnancy in agonadal women – which has been the subject of much medico-legal debate recently. The majority of the data reviewed are unpublished or have been published during the last 5 years, and were generated in relation to women who, according to the various authors, had undergone a premature menopause, either natural or surgical. It is not clear whether the results apply equally to women with primary ovarian failure causing primary amenorrhoea, and caution must be exercised with any extrapolation.

Consequences of ovarian failure

As with natural or surgical menopause around age 50 years, these can be divided into short and long-term.

Short-term consequences: Various authors[2-7] have commented upon the presence of hot flushes and genital tract atrophy in women with premature ovarian failure; the majority of the studies reported that these symptoms were present in fewer than 50% of patients. However, some of these studies included patients with 'resistant ovary syndrome' and auto-immune forms of ovarian disease from which a minority of patients obviously recovered fully because pregnancy later occurred! Additionally, none of the studies attempted to determine, in detail, the impact of symptomatology on sexual function, nor on femininity or social behaviour. We believe such additional information to be of value in clinical management.

To provide this information and to ensure, as best we could, that our patients did not have ovarian function, we conducted a study in teenage girls and women who had undergone treatment for acute myeloid leukaemia (AML). All had received total body irradiation (TBI) prior to bone marrow transplantation (BMT), and because the ovary is a well recognised site for metastatic disease, no attempt had been made to shield the gonads during irradiation. None subsequently regained ovarian function.

The study group comprised 29 patients, the majority of whom were interviewed by one of us (MIW), and they were then sent a purpose-designed questionnaire which was sub-divided so as to obtain information on:

(1) the frequency of classic, oestrogen-deficiency symptoms (flushes, sweats and vaginal dryness),
(2) anxieties about sterility and appearance, feelings of loss of femininity, and worries about loss of menstruation,
(3) whether ovarian failure had changed social habits, and
(4) the frequency of sexual difficulties.

Nineteen patients (66%) responded; their mean age was 27.2 years (range 14–41 years), and the mean duration since TBI and BMT was 3.5 years (range 6 months–6 years).

The results are summarised in Table 6.1. Twelve (63%) of the nineteen patients reported hot flushes; although numbers are small, there was no age-dependent effect and the teenagers and 30–39 year old women were similarly affected. Identical comments apply to night sweats. Two of the 3 patients *NOT* reporting vaginal dryness were non-sexually active teenagers (14 and 16 years old).

As expected, the majority of patients concerned about sterility were nulliparous. Interestingly, 8 of the nine patients worried about their appearance complained of dry skin and hair. These symptoms are commonly reported by middle-aged women after natural menopause, and are then often ascribed to oestrogen deficiency. However, we believe that caution must be exercised in assuming the same aetiology in this study group; the adverse effects on skin and hair might have been caused by the radiotherapy. Seven patients felt a loss of femininity, and 9 patients reported that their social life had been adversely affected. These problems tended to occur in patients under 25 years old.

Table 6.1 TOTAL NUMBER OF PATIENTS (PERCENTAGE) REPORTING PROBLEM

Hot flushes	12 (63%)
Night Sweats	7 (36%)
Vaginal Dryness	16 (84%)
Worry about:	
Sterility	9 (47%)
Appearance	9 (47%)
Menstruation (loss of)	4 (21%)
Loss of Femininity	7 (37%)
Adverse effects of social life	9 (47%)

Fourteen of the 19 patients were sexually active prior to TBI and BMT; subsequently, 12 reported difficulties with intercourse leading to loss of interest, and 11 reported difficulty in achieving orgasm. Two women become anorgasmic and apareunic in their early thirties.

Long-term consequences:
Osteoporosis. The debate on whether ageing or natural menopause is the more important determinant of postmenopausal bone loss has continued for many years. For women undergoing menopause around age 50 years, prospective studies have shown a discernible decrease in radial bone mass at this time[8]. Comparable, prospective data for trabecular bone are not currently available because, quite simply, the required studies have not yet been performed. Cross-sectional data on vertebral density have yielded conflicting results. Some studies have suggested linear models to describe the changes in vertebral mass from age 20 years to over 70 years[9]; others have indicated more complex models with a peak in the mid-thirties followed by an accelerating decline through to age 80 years[10]; most recently, it has been observed that perimenopausal women appear to show more rapid vertebral bone loss than their pre or postmenopausal counterparts[11].

If, because of a lack of prospective data, there is no consensus on the effects of natural menopause around age 50 years on the vertebral bone mass, then it is hardly surprising that an identical situation exists for premature natural menopause. Indeed, there are also no data from prospective, controlled studies available to determine the effects of premature natural menopause on cortical bone. This lack of information may, initially, appear surprising given that the first reports linking premature menopause (albeit surgical) to an increased incidence of osteoporotic fractures (mainly of the distal radius) were published in the mid 1970s[12]. However, premature natural menopause occurs sporadically and, in our experience, the majority of patients with the condition do not seek medical advice for many months after cessation of menses; additionally, the condition is not that common. The costs of screening a premenopausal population (essential for baseline values) which is large enough to produce women who subsequently undergo premature natural menopause in numbers adequate for meaningful studies are prohibitive. Lack of adequate numbers of women with premature natural menopause almost certainly explains why no large-scale retrospective studies have been published on incidence rates for the classic osteoporotic fractures in this group.

At present, therefore, we have to rely on cross-sectional studies to provide information on the effects of early loss of ovarian function, and the majority of such studies have investigated castrates. There are potential disadvantages with this type of study group because it is not known whether rates of bone loss are similar after surgical and premature natural menopause, and it is usually assumed that the condition requiring surgery did not interfere with the sex hormone environment and thereby affect bone mass. Despite this limitation, data are available which clearly indicate that premature surgical menopause is associated with reduced bone mass.

Some of the results from the study of Richelson et al[13] are illustrated in Figure 6.1. To determine the relative contributions of ageing and oestrogen deficiency to postmenopausal bone loss, 3 groups, each of 14 women, were studied. The 'premature menopause' group had a mean age of 54 years and all patients had undergone oophorectomy during young adulthood; the mean duration of oestrogen deficiency was 22 years. The 'perimenopausal group' of similar mean age, 52 years, served as 'controls', and the mean interval since natural menopause was 0.3 years. An older natural 'postmenopausal group' had a mean age of 73 years but an identical mean time since menopause (22 years) as compared to the premature menopause group. The bone mineral density at 4 skeletal sites for these 3 groups is as shown: as compared to the perimenopausal group, bone mineral density was significantly lower in both the premature menopause and older postmenopausal groups at all 4 skeletal sites ($p < 0.05 - p < 0.001$); these differences, expressed as percentages, are as shown in Table 6.2. However, there were no significant differences in bone mineral density at any site between the premature and older postmenopausal groups. Interestingly, vertebral wedge compression fractures were seen on roentgenograms in 2 patients in the premature menopausal and in 2 patients in the older postmenopausal groups.

Arterial Disease. It is often stated that menopause is a major determinant of arterial disease, and particularly coronary heart disease (CHD) in women. We find this difficult to justify from the literature. For example, Colditz et al[14] recently cited 11 studies in which age-adjusted rates of CHD were observed to increase after menopause; they also cited 8 studies which failed to demonstrate such an association.

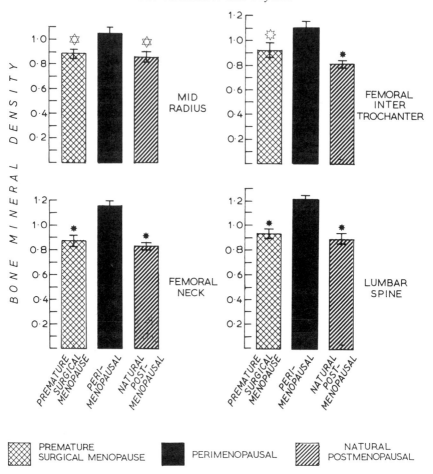

FIGURE 6.1 Bone mineral density at four skeletal sites in three groups of women: see text for details of groups.
* $p < 0.01$ for premature surgical menopause and natural post-menopause groups as
* $p < 0.001$ compared with the perimenopausal group.
* $p < 0.5$

Reproduced, with permission, from Richelson et al. (1984) *New England Journal of Medicine*, **311**, 1273–1275

It must be remembered that both age and the degree of cigarette consumption are important predictors of CHD[15]. The importance of the former is illustrated in Figure 6.2, which shows annual death rates for CHD in the USA in 1979. Between the ages of 30–34 years and 40–44 years, the rate increased approximately 8–9 fold in women; between the latter and ages 50–54 years, there was a further 4-fold increase. Since natural menopause is highly correlated with age, and is also influenced by cigarette consumption, a spurious association between natural menopause and CHD may be observed unless these confounding variables are taken into account.

Table 6.2 PERCENTAGE DIFFERENCE IN BONE MINERAL DENSITY BETWEEN THE PREMATURE SURGICAL MENOPAUSE AND NATURAL POSTMENOPAUSE GROUPS AS COMPARED TO THE PERIMENOPAUSAL GROUP.

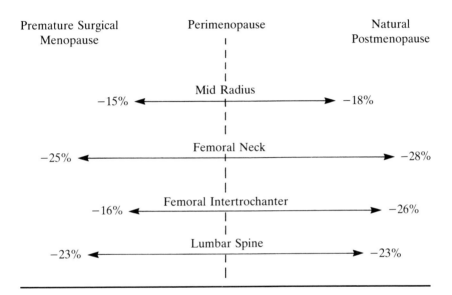

Adapted from Richelson et al. (1984) *New England Journal of Medicine*, 311, 1273–1275 and used with permission.

If the precise relationship between CHD and natural menopause around aged 50 years has not been fully elucidated, what of that between CHD and premature surgical menopause? For reasons stated previously, the majority of studies investigating the effects of premature menopause on CHD risk have used castrates. It is now almost 30 years since Oliver and Boyd[16] first reported that castration increases the risk of CHD, and numerous similar reports soon followed[12,17]. It is easy, now, to criticise these early papers because of imprecise methodology, lack of appropriate control groups in some instances, and small numbers. However, the recent publication of a large, prospective study has confirmed these original observations.

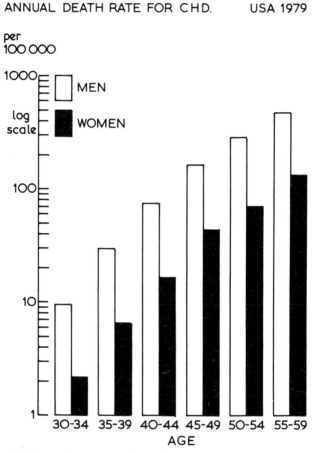

FIGURE 6.2   Death rates for coronary heart disease for men and women, ages 30–59, in the United States in 1979.

Colditz et al[14] analysed data on a prospective cohort of 127,000 American women aged 30–35 years who were followed from 1976 to 1982. Appropriate information was obtained in 1976 and was updated by mailing questionnaires every 2 years; the accuracy of the collected data was validated. The risk of CHD according to type of menopause is as shown in Table 6.3, adjusted for age and smoking. Natural menopause and hysterectomy with or without unilateral oophorectomy were not associated with an increase in risk of CHD (rate ratios 1.2 and 1.0, respectively). However, women who had undergone bilateral oophorectomy had an increased risk (rate ratio 2.2). These authors also evaluated the effects of postmenopausal oestrogen therapy. As compared with premenopausal women, natural menopause together with oestrogen use did not affect the risk (rate ratio 0.8). Oestrogen use in the castrates appeared to eliminate the increase among these women as compared to premenopausal women (rate ratio 0.9).

Table 6.3 RISK OF CORONARY HEART DISEASE, ADJUSTED FOR AGE AND SMOK-ING, ACCORDING TO TYPE OF MENOPAUSE AND POSTMENOPAUSAL ESTROGEN THERAPY, ESTIMATED FROM PROPORTIONAL-HAZARDS ANALYSIS

Type of menopause	*Rate ratio (95% confidence limits)*	
	Untreated	*Oestrogen users*
* Natural menopause	1.2 (0.8, 1.8)	0.8 (0.4, 1.3)
**Hysterectomy ± unilateral oophorectomy	1.0 (0.3, 2.6)	1.8 (0.8, 3.8)
**Hysterectomy + bilateral oophorectomy	2.2 (1.2, 4.2)	0.9 (0.6, 1.6)

* Controlling for age in one-year intervals: smoking as current, past or never; and follow-up interval, 1976–78, 1978–80 or 1980–82.
**Controlling for age in five-year intervals: smoking as current, past or never; and follow-up interval, 1976–78, 1978–80, or 1980–82.
Adapted from Colditz et al. (1987) *New England Journal of Medicine,* **316**, 1105–1110 and reproduced with permission.

Pregnancy in agonadal women

In countries with sympathetic religious beliefs, artificial insemination by donor (AID), which was first described in 1884[18], has been an acceptable treatment for many years for couples in which the male is infertile. The converse, the establishment of a pregnancy in a couple in whom the wife is infertile, was not reported until 1983[19], and the first report of a successful pregnancy with delivery of a healthy baby in a woman with premature ovarian failure appeared one year later[20].

Although medically analogous to sperm donation, oocyte donation is technically much more demanding because it requires methods for monitoring follicular development and oocyte retrieval; subsequent pre-requisites for pregnancy are fertilisation *in vitro* and embryo dona-tion into a receptive endometrium. Further considerations in agonadal patients are the maintenance of the pregnancy by exogenous hormones until steroidogenesis by the feto-placental unit is sufficient to prevent abortion, and finally, the method of delivery. Pregnancy maintenance has been reviewed in detail recently[21], and will not be considered here. It suffices to say that exogenous hormones can maintain pregnancy until steroid production by the feto-placental unit is adequate. Too few data are currently available to comment sensibly upon the necessity for caesarian section in women with premature menopause. In a patient with premature ovarian failure and primary amenorrhoea, Lutjen et al[22] commented upon the hard, undilated cervix and short, inner uterine segment at caesarian section at 40 weeks gestation. Whether these unfavourable features were due to too early resort to surgery or due to little or no exposure to ovarian steroids during early post-pubertal development is not known.

The historical aspects of *in vitro* fertilisation (IVF) and embryo donation, and the results of experimentation in other mammalian species have recently been the subject of an extensive review[21], to which the interested reader is referred. In man, the techniques for fertilisation *in vitro* are now so well established that they need not be considered further here. Similar comments apply to super-ovulation; successful regimens have been developed and more than 4 oocytes can be recovered from the majority of patients in many conventional IVF programmes. The mean number of oocytes recovered per cycle in our IVF programme at King's during the last 12 months has exceeded seven. Thus, the problems currently encountered by those who run oocyte donation and IVF programmes are not technical, they are social, ethical and legal.

Oocyte donation

In theory, any woman not affected by an inherited disorder who has ovaries which respond appropriately to gonadotrophin stimulation and which are accessible for oocyte recovery *can* donate oocytes. However, the critical question as far as the legislators are concerned is who *should be allowed* to donate oocytes? Should donation be permitted between relatives, between known donors, or should it always be anonymous? Longer-term issues have been the legal status of the child, and whether he/she should have the right to discover the identity of the genetic mother.

In addition to pioneering the technical aspects of IVF and embryo donation, the Australians were also the first to introduce appropriate legislation. The Waller Committee, appointed by the Victorian Government in 1982, supported the use of donor oocytes from both known and anonymous donors[23], and the first report of the establishment of a pregnancy after oocyte donation between relatives (sisters) appeared in 1986[24]. The Victorian Parliament passed the Status of Children (Amendment) Act in 1984[25]; this gave full legal status to the recipient woman.

To date, most other countries have not legislated. Some, such as the United Kingdom, have established independent authorities which issue licences to medical centres which adhere to the authority's guide lines. The Voluntary Licensing Authority (VLA) in the United Kingdom has approved anonymous oocyte donation, but has stated that donation between known donors or relatives 'should be carried out only under exceptional circumstances'[26]. We can understand the *preference* of the VLA for anonymous donation. In one of the few studies of attitudes of patients who underwent conventional IVF and who donated oocytes, Leeton and Harman[27] reported that 31 of their 34 patients (91%) preferred to donate anonymously. Some of their data[27] are reproduced in Table 6.4. Interestingly, 16 patients (47%) were prepared to donate to a known recipient; of these, 6 patients (18%) were prepared to donate to a relative, 2 (6%) to a close friend, and 8 women (24%) were prepared to donate to either.

We believe that donation between friends and relatives should be permitted if both parties have been appropriately counselled and are agreeable. The supply of oocytes donated by patients undergoing conventional IVF cannot meet the current demand and, in our opinion, this supply is threatened; the more widespread introduction of embryo freezing will drastically reduce the number of spare oocytes available for donation. Alternative sources of donor oocytes will have to be found. The value of patients undergoing gamete intra-fallopian transfer (GIFT) is likely to be limited because of greater availability of embryo freezing. Patients undergoing laparoscopic sterilisation are an attractive alternative, but our experience of trying to recruit them has been very disappointing. Letters were mailed to 50 women awaiting sterilisation at King's College Hospital asking whether they would donate oocytes; only 2 responded positively. If alternative sources cannot be found to meet the demand, then we believe that a 'black market' may well be created and the pioneering recommendation of the Ethics Committee of The American Fertility Society[28], which discouraged payment to donors, will have been in vain.

Table 6.4 ATTITUDE OF DONOR TO RECIPIENT

Question	Answer	Number
Would you object if your egg was used to allow a married/single woman to have a child?	Married woman	
	Yes	0
	No	34 (100%)
	Single woman	
	Yes	22 (65%)
	No	10 (29%)
	Uncertain	2 (6%)
Would you wish to choose the parents?	Yes	3 (9%)
	No	31 (91%)
Would you wish to meet the mother?	Yes	2 (6%)
	No	30 (88%)
	Uncertain	2(6%)
Would you donate to a known recipient?	Yes	16 (47%)
	No	18 (53%)
If yes, would you prefer to donate to either		
a relative	Yes	6
a close friend	Yes	2
	Either	8

Reproduced, with permission, from Leeton and Harman (1986) *Journal of In Vitro Fertilization and Embryo Transfer*, **3**, 374– 378

Endometrial priming and embryo transfer

The available data in both men and monkeys have recently been extensively reviewed[21], and will only be briefly summarised here. Oestrogens have been given orally[19,20,22], and intra-vaginally[21]; progesterone has been administered intra-vaginally[19,20], intra-muscularly[29], and orally (our unpublished observations). The schedule that resulted in the first successful pregnancy in a woman with premature menopause is reproduced in Figure 6.3[20]. Oestradiol valerate (Progynova: Schering) was taken orally at 24 hourly intervals at doses of 1 or 2 mg per day (days 1–9 and 14–28), or at 8 hourly intervals at a dose of 6 mg per day (days 10–13). Progesterone was administered as a single 25 or 50 mg intra-vaginal pessary once a day (days 15–16), or 2 pessaries introduced separately at 12 hourly intervals (days 17–26).

With many of the current schedules, asynchrony in epithelial glandular and stromal maturation has been observed in the first half of the luteal phase[21]. Despite this, the endometrium is clearly receptive to donated embryos and by the Spring of 1987, approximately 30 pregnancies had been reported in the worldwide literature[20-22,29-34]. Only an approximate number can be given because not all authors have clearly stated whether the recipients were suffering from premature menopause, or other forms of infertility necessitating ovum donation and IVF. The number of pregnancies, to date, is too small for meaningful comparisons between the treatment regimens. Despite the paucity of the data, the experience of Rosenwaks[21] suggests that the optimal timing of embryo donation is between days 17–19 of the cycle as compared to days 20–24. With the former, Rosenwaks[21] reported that all 7 patients receiving embryos became pregnant; none of the 7 patients in whom embryos were transferred on day 20 or later conceived.

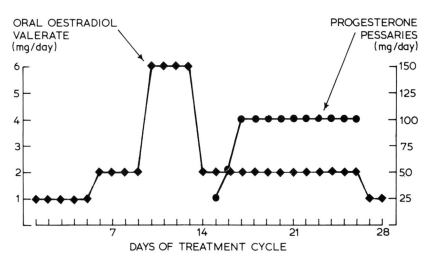

FIGURE 6.3 Dose regimen for the cyclic replacement of oestrogen and progesterone. Reproduced, with permission, from Lutjen et al. (1984). *Nature*, **307**, 174–175

Summary and conclusions

It has not been the aim of this chapter to provide a comprehensive review of all aspects of premature menopause but to comment, for the specialist and non-specialist, upon various aspects of the topic in which new data have been published during the last 5 years. Progressive specialisation, an inevitable accompaniment of research, has draw-backs. The infertility specialist establishing an IVF and embryo dona-tion programme may have little knowledge of the long-term effects of ovarian failure upon bone and arterial status, and the menopause specialist may be unaware that pregnancy success is increasingly being achieved with IVF and embryo donation.

Our understanding of the short and long-term consequences of ova-rian failure is incomplete. There are no large scale studies on the effects of premature, natural menopause, and this is due, we believe, to the sporadic occurrence of the condition and to the obvious difficul-ties in obtaining baseline (premenopausal) data. Thus, most workers to date have tended to investigate castrates but caution must be exercised in extrapolating data from the latter to women undergoing premature natural menopause. With improved cytotoxic and radiotherapy techni-ques, increasing numbers of girls and women with haemopoietic dis-eases, such as leukaemia, will survive but they will be agonadal. They provide another source of patients for study purposes and our pre-liminary data (Table 6.1) confirm previous reports[2-7] that the majority of women with premature menopause experience flushes, sweats and vaginal dryness. In our study, the latter was particularly troublesome and caused sexual difficulties in approximately 80% of previously sexually-active girls and women. Although patient numbers are small, there was a trend for the major sexual problems to be associated with a withdrawal from social activities – particularly in patients under 25 years old. Previous studies have failed to investigate the impact of ovarian failure upon appearance and feminine identity; our data sug-gest an appreciable impact but we stress that it is not clear if the dry skin and hair, which were commonly reported, were due to radiother-apy or oestrogen deficiency. More data are urgently required so that appropriate treatment and counselling may be initiated before irrever-sible physical and psychological damage results. This is particularly important because the numbers of leukaemics, who are cured, will increase.

Fortunately, data are available from well-conducted, prospective stu-dies on the effects of early loss of ovarian function (castration) on bone density[13] (Figure 6.1; Table 6.2), and on the risk of CHD[14] (Table 6.3). The former study has clearly demonstrated that early castration significantly reduces bone density at various skeletal sites, and that cortical and trabecular bone are affected. The risk of fracture is likely to be increased correspondingly. The largest, prospective study published to date has demonstrated that surgical menopause doubles the risk of CHD[14]. These data are even more alarming when the frequency of CHD is considered; it is the number one cause of death in Western countries and any condition which increases the risk substantially will have important implications for health care resources. Thus, it seems imperative to prescribe effective therapy to agonadal women to prevent the development of the serious short and long-term consequences of ovarian failure at an unacceptable age.

Quite deliberately, we have refrained from discussing oestrogen therapy in this review. In middle-aged women who have undergone natural menopause, there are insufficient data to draw meaningful conclusions as to whether oral or parenteral oestrogens (transdermal, percutaneous, subcutaneous, intramuscular and intravaginal) are more beneficial with respect to arterial status[35]. No data addressing this specific issue are available for women with premature menopause, although it is clear that oral oestrogens can prevent the increase in risk which follows castration[14] (Table 6.3). At appropriate doses, oral, percutaneous and subcutaneously administered oestrogens have been shown to conserve both cortical and trabecular bone in middle-aged women who have undergone natural menopause, and we see no reason why similar benefits will not occur following premature surgical or natural menopause. At present, the transdermal systems have not been available for long enough for effective bone conservation to be demonstrated; however, it is clear that these systems cause the biochemical changes associated with skeletal protection. Similarly, whilst it is clear that progestogens should be added in women with an intact uterus, the optimal type and dose of progestogen, and duration of administration, remain controversial[36]. Because of financial considerations, should young agonadal women receive conventional hormone replacement therapy, or the oral contraceptive pill? The recently introduced triphasic contraceptives have a beneficial impact on lipid and lipoprotein metabolism[37]; however, it is not known whether they increase the risk of venous thrombotic disease.

Infertility, perhaps the most damaging consequence of early loss of ovarian function, can now be overcome. The medical aspects of oocyte donation, in terms of ovarian hyperstimulation and oocyte recovery, are well established. The legal aspects, however, have not been addressed by most countries, and international laws do not exist. Who should be allowed to donate? With the demand for oocytes exceeding the supply, should payment to the donor be outlawed? What is the legal status of the child? Should the child have the right to discover the identity of the genetic mother? Unless these issues are addressed quickly, chaos is likely to ensue because it can be confidently predicted that the number of Units running successful IVF and embryo donation programmes will increase dramatically during the next 5 years. Australia no longer has the monopoly and pregnancies have been reported in Austria, Belgium, Italy, the United Kingdom and the United States.

Many more data are required on the optimal management of the recipient. Various regimens for endometrial priming have been described[19-22,24,29-34], but no comparative studies exist. Will alterations to the 'priming' regimens increase the pregnancy rate? Similar comments apply to the optimal timing of embryo donation – although the preliminary data of Rosenwaks[21] strongly suggest that embryo donation on days 17–19 of the cycle is more effective than on days 20–24.

Finally, what will be the medical consequences of banning ovum donation between friends and/or relatives, and relying solely on anonymous donation? With the former, the cycle of the recipient can easily be synchronised with that of the donor. However, with anonymous donation, this will not be possible; the recipient will be on oestrogen/progestogen therapy but a suitable oocyte may not become available when the endometrium is receptive. Two alternatives are available to overcome this problem. The first is embryo freezing and subsequent thawing for embryo donation at the appropriate time[31]. However, for reasons discussed earlier, we believe that embryo freezing will reduce the supply of oocytes for donation. The second strategy is hormone manipulation of the recipient to advance or retard the endometrium – as appropriate – so that the embryo can be transferred at the optimal time. It remains to be determined whether this can be achieved.

We now know a great deal more about some of the consequences of premature menopause and about various aspects of treatment than we did 5 years ago, but we still know very little.

Acknowledgements

We thank Dr R. Powles, MD, BSc, FRCP, Physician in Charge, Leukaemia Unit, Royal Marsden Hospital, Sutton, Surrey and Dr. Myra Hunter B.A., Dip. Clin. Psych., Clinical Psychologist, King's

College Hospital for all their help. The assistance of Miss J. Bennett in the preparation of this manuscript, and of the Imperial Cancer Research Fund, Lincoln's Inn Fields, WC2A 3PX to M. I. Whitehead is gratefully acknowledged.

REFERENCES

1. Coulam, C. B. (ed.) (1983). Premature gonadal failure. In: *Seminars in Reproductive Endocrinology*, **1, No. 2**, (New York: Thieme-Stratton)
2. Russell, P., Bannatyne, P., Shearman, R. P. et al. (1982). Premature hypergonadotropic ovarian failure: clinicopathological study of 19 cases. *International Journal of Gynecological Pathology*, **1**, 185
3. Board, J. A., Redwine, F. O., Moncure, C. W. et al. (1979). Identification of differing etiologies of clinically diagnosed premature menopause. *American Journal of Obstetrics and Gynecology*, **134**, 936
4. Rebar, R. W., Erickson, G. F. and Yen, S. S. C. (1982). Idiopathic premature ovarian failure: clinical and endocrine characteristics. *Fertility and Sterility*, **37**, 35
5. Zarate, A., Karchmer, S., Gomez, E., et al. (1970). Premature menopause. A clinical, histological and cytogenetic study. *American Journal of Obstetrics and Gynecology*, **106**, 110
6. Keettel, W. C. and Bradbury, J. T. (1964). Premature ovarian failure, permanent and temporary. *American Journal of Obstetrics and Gynecology*, **89**, 83
7. Aiman, J. and Smentek, C. (1985). Premature ovarian failure. *Obstetrics and Gynecology*, **66**, 9–14
8. Hui, S. L., Wiske, P. S., Norton, J. A. and Johnston, C. C. Jr. (1982). A prospective study of change in bone mass with age in postmenopausal women. *Journal of Chronic Diseases*, **35**, 715– 725
9. Riggs, B. L., Wahner, H. W., Dunn, W. L., Mazess, R. B., Offord, K. P. and Melton, L. J. III. (1981). Differential changes in bone mineral density of the appendicular and axial skeleton with aging: relationship to spinal osteoporosis. *Journal of Clinical Investigation*, **67**, 328–335
10. Krolner, B. and Nielsen, S. P. (1982). Bone mineral content of the lumbar spine in normal and osteoporotic women: cross-sectional and longitudinal studies. *Clinical Science*, **62**, 329–336
11. Hui, S. L., Slemenda, C. W., Johnston, C. C. and Appledorn, C. R. (1987). Effects of age and menopause on vertebral bone density. *Bone and Mineral*, **2**, 141–146
12. Johansson, B. W., Kaij, L., Kullander, S., Lenner, H-C., Svanberg, L. and Astedt, B. (1975). On some late effects of bilateral oophorectomy in the age range 15–30 years. *Acta Obstetricia et Gynecologica Scandinavica*, **54**, 449–461

13. Richelson, L. S., Wahner, H. W., Melton, L. J. III, and Riggs, B. L. (1984). Relative contributions of aging and estrogen deficiency to postmenopausal bone loss. *New England Journal of Medicine*, **311**, 1273–1275

14. Colditz, G. A., Willett, W. C., Stampfer, M. J., Rosner, B., Speizer, F. E. and Hennekens, C. H. (1987). Menopause and the risk of coronary heart disease in women. *New England Journal of Medicine*, **316**, 1105–1110

15. Bush, T. L., Barrett-Connor, E., Cowan, L. D., Criqui, M. H., Wallace, R. B., Suchindran, C. H., Tyroler, H. A. and Rifkind, B. A. (1987). Cardiovascular mortality and non-contraceptive use of estrogens in women: results from the Lipid Research Center Program Follow-up Study. *Circulation*, **75**, 1102–1109

16. Oliver, M. F. and Boyd, G. S. (1959). Effect of bilateral ovariectomy on coronary-artery disease and serum-lipid levels. *Lancet*, **2**, 690–694

17. Sznajderman, M. and Oliver, M. F. (1963). Spontaneous premature menopause ischaemic heart-disease, and serum-lipids. *Lancet*, **1**, 962–965

18. Finegold, W. (1976). In: *Artificial Insemination*, p.7. (Springfield, Illinois: Charles C. Thomas)

19. Trounson, A., Leeton, J., Besanko, M., Wood, C. and Conti, A. (1983). Pregnancy established in an infertile patient after transfer of a donated embryo fertilised in vitro. *British Medical Journal*, **286**, 835–838

20. Lutjen, P., Trounson, A., Leeton, J., Findley, J., Wood, C. and Renou, P. (1984). The establishment and maintenance of pregnancy using in vitro fertilisation and embryo donation in a patient with primary ovarian failure. *Nature*, **307**, 174–175

21. Rosenwaks, Z. (1987). Donor eggs: their application in modern reproductive technologies. *Fertility and Sterility*, **47**, 895–909

22. Lutjen, P., Leeton, J., Trounson, A., Renou, P., Wood, C. and Findley, J. (1985). Pregnancy without ovarian function. *Journal of in Vitro Fertilisation and Embryo Transfer*, **2**, 107–108

23. The Committee to Consider the Social, Ethical and Legal Issues Arising from In Vitro Fertilisation: Report on Donor Gametes. (1983). (Victoria. Australia: Law Reform Department), p.22

24. Leeton, J., Chan, L. K., Trounson, A. and Harman, J. (1986). Pregnancy established in an infertile patient after transfer of an embryo fertilised in vitro where the oocyte was donated by the sister of the recipient. *Journal of in Vitro Fertilisation and Embryo Transfer*, **3**, 379–382

25. Victorian Parliament: Status of Children (Amendment) Act. (1984). (Melbourne: Victorian Government Print Office)

26. The First Report of the Voluntary Licencing Authority for Human In Vitro Fertilisation and Embryology. (1986). p.15

27. Leeton, J. and Harman, J. (1986). Attitudes toward egg donation of thirty-four infertile women who donated during their in vitro fertilisation treatment. *Journal of in Vitro Fertilisation and Embryo Transfer*, **3**, 374–378

28. The Ethics Committee of The American Fertility Society: Ethical consid-

erations of the new reproductive technologies. (1986). *Fertility and Sterility*, **4** (suppl. 1), 1S

29. Navot, D., Laufer, N., Kopolovic, J., Rabinowitz, R., Birkenfeld, A., Lewin, A., Granat, M., Margaliot, E. and Shenker, J. G. (1986). Artificially induced endometrial cycles and establishment of pregnancies in the absence of ovaries. *New England Journal of Medicine*, **314**, 806

30. Feichtinger, W. and Kemeter, P. (1985). Pregnancy after total ovariectomy achieved by ovum donation. *Lancet*, **2**, 722

31. Devroey, P., Braeckmans, P., Camus, M., Khan, I., Smitz, J., Staessens, C., van der Abbeel, E., van Waesberghe, L., Wisanto, A. and van Steirteghan, A. C. (1987). Pregnancies after replacement of fresh and frozen-thawed embryos in a donation program. In: W. Feichtinger and P. Kemeter (eds). *Future Aspects of Human in Vitro Fertilization*, p.133. (Berlin: Springer-Verlag)

32. Lutjen, P., Healy, D., Chan, C., Leeton, J. and Trounson, A. (1986). The Australian method of embryo and oocyte donation. *Journal of in Vitro Fertilisation and Embryo Transfer*, **3**, 69 (abstract 19)

33. Lejeune, B., Englert, Y., Puissant, F., Camus, M., Dehou, M. F. and Leroy, F. (1986). Pregnancy obtained by oocyte donation, in vitro fertilisation and embryo transfer in a case of primary ovarian failure. *Journal of in Vitro Fertilisation and Embryo Transfer*, **3**, 70 (abstract 20)

34. Gianaroli, L., Ferraretti, A. P., Bianchi, L., Violini, F., Montacuti, V. and Flamigni, C. (1986). Establishment of pregnancies after in vitro fertilisation of donated oocytes in infertile women. *Journal of in Vitro Fertilisation and Embryo Transfer*, **3**, 179 (abstract 209)

35. Whitehead, M. I. and Fraser, D. (1987). Controversies concerning the safety of estrogen replacement therapy. *American Journal of Obstetrics and Gynecology*, **156**, 1313–1322

36. Whitehead, M. I. and Fraser, D. (1987). The effects of estrogens and progestogens on the endometrium: modern approach to treatment. In: D. R. Gambrell (ed). *Obstetrics and Gynecology Clinics of North America*, 14, 1, pp. 299–320

37. Shargil, A. A. and Sharff, A. A. (1983). Estrogen replacement in menopause and bone mass, osteoarthritis, calcium balance and lipid metabolism. In: *XI Meeting of the International Study Group for Steroid Hormones*. Vol. 2 (2)

SECTION 2

Workshop reports

7

Overview of the concept of the andropause

Chairman: L. GOOREN (NETHERLANDS)
Speakers: L. Gooren (Netherlands)
R. Rubens (Belgium)

The andropause or decline in sexual function in the aging male is a puzzling problem. Some 2000 years ago *Cicero* wrote: "Ut non omne virum, sic non omnis aetas vetustate coacescit". It is well-known that the menopause marks the end of reproductive life in the female, but a similar sharp end point is generally not seen in males. However, despite great variability, the clinical, histological and biochemical data converge towards the conclusion that there is a male climacteric.

Secondary sex characteristics

Androgen-dependent body-hair growth decreases in the elderly male[1]. Furthermore, the prevalence of gynaecomastia in males above the age of 45 exceeds 50%[2], being significantly greater than in young men.

Potency and libido

The elderly male is less vigorous in his sex life, even in the presence of a very attractive partner, a fact that has been documented since biblical time[3]. The cross-sectional study carried out by Martin[4] showed clearly decreased sexual activity in the aging male. However, since neurological and vascular diseases are very common in elderly males, it is difficult, by means of epidemiological cross-sectional studies, to distinguish secondary impotence due to underlying diseases from essential or primary impotence due to old age itself.

Testicular morphology

Using a Prader orchidometer, a decrease in testicular volume was observed by various groups[5,6].

Decreased testicular weight is due mainly to a lowering of the parenchymal weight in conjunction with an increase in tunica weight[7]. A histological change is apparent within the testicle, with a thickening of the basal membranes, narrowing of the tubular lumen and a simultaneous alteration in the testicular vasculature[8].

Sperm production and fertility

Blum[9] was the first to report the increase in the prevalence of azoospermia in the sixth to eighth decades of life.

Different investigators[10,11] have reported a decrease in sperm motility and morphology with increasing age.

Johnson et al.[12] have reported a decrease in daily sperm production in old age, as assessed by post-mortem examinations.

Owing to marital patterns, fertility in old age is very difficult to assess. On the other hand, different reports have documented maintained fertility in old age[13], although a decrease in fertility with increasing age was apparent in population studies[14].

Endocrine changes in elderly males

Total testosterone plasma levels in elderly males: Few data concerning plasma testosterone in elderly males appeared in the literature prior to 1972. In that year, using a very reliable gas-liquid chromatography method we were able to show[15] a decrease in plasma testosterone from the seventh decade of life onwards.

Other investigators[16,17] confirmed these results during the following year. We ourselves tested the same hypothesis again a year later[18] using a radioimmunoassay (RIA) method and confirmed our original observations. The results were subsequently reconfirmed in different countries.

However, in 1980 a number of reports[19–21] did not document any decrease in androgen levels in old age.

A new investigation was performed in our laboratory. A population sample living in exceptionally constant circumstances (Benedictine monks) was investigated, using rigorously strict methods. A decrease in plasma testosterone levels was again observed in this population[22]. The study was later extended to a normal suburban community, all data were obtained under standardized conditions and the results proved to be very similar to the 1972 findings (Figure 7.1).

Free testosterone, testosterone binding globulin (TeBG) and metabolic clearance rate: It is generally assumed that free testosterone is the only part of the testosterone circulating in plasma that is biologically active. As the TeBG concentration increases with age (Figure 7.2) a decrease is seen in free testosterone (from 10.3 ± 3.5 ng/dl at age 20–30 to 2.6 ± 1.3 ng/dl after age 80)[15].

The metabolic clearance rate of testosterone is slightly decreased, resulting in a net decrease in the blood production rate (6.6 mg/24 hours in young as against 3.9 mg/24 hours in elderly males)[15].

Human chorionic gonadotrophin (HCG) stimulation: To assess the reserve capacity of the testicular endocrine function, the response of the testosterone level to an exogenous stimulus such as HCG has been studied[18].

It can be seen from Figure 7.3 that although testosterone secretion increases in elderly males, the absolute levels remain lower than those in young adults.

These data suggest that the Leydig cells retain a reserve capacity which, although diminished, remains active.

Gonadotrophins and luteinizing hormone releasing hormone (LHRH): In post-menopausal women an increase in gonadotrophins occurs concomitantly with the decrease in ovarian function. We have previously reported an increase in the level of gonadotrophins with advancing age in elderly men[15]. These findings have been confirmed by all authors. Zumoff et al.[23] reported an unchanged luteinizing hormone (LH), but an increased follicle-stimulating hormone (FSH) level in elderly males.

Recently, Warner et al.[24] have published data on bioassayable LH which are discrepant with the increased immunoassayable LH in old men. The decrease in bioassayable LH could explain the decrease in testosterone levels in the presence of increased immunoassayable LH in aging men.

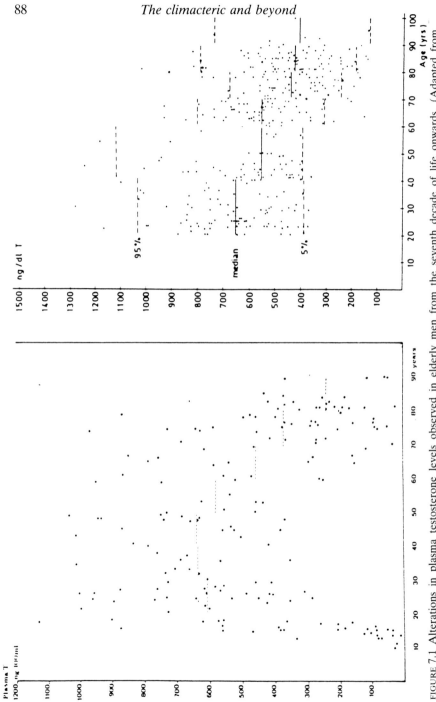

FIGURE 7.1 Alterations in plasma testosterone levels observed in elderly men from the seventh decade of life onwards. (Adapted from Vermeulen and Rubens, 1972[15] and from Deslypere and Vermeulen, 1984[22].)

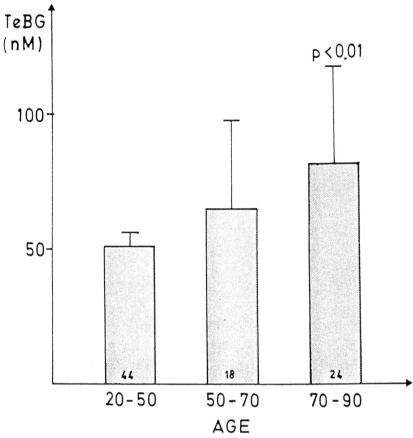

FIGURE 7.2 Testosterone binding globulin (TeBG) concentration at various ages.

It was recently demonstrated that the number of LH pulses, which reflects hypothalamic LHRH release, decreases in old age[25]. This indicates that aging affects not only the testis but also the hypothalamus.

Gooren et al.[26] recently demonstrated that aging men respond more readily to an oestrogen stimulus with a positive feedback of LH. Younger men do so only after prolonged oestrogen exposure. This again indicates that the aging process also affects neuroendocrine functions.

To test the pituitary reserve, an LHRH stimulation study was performed. Although the peak values were higher in the elderly group, the proportional increase was more pronounced in the younger group[18]. Similar results have been reported by Harman et al.[27].

HCG   1500 IM/day

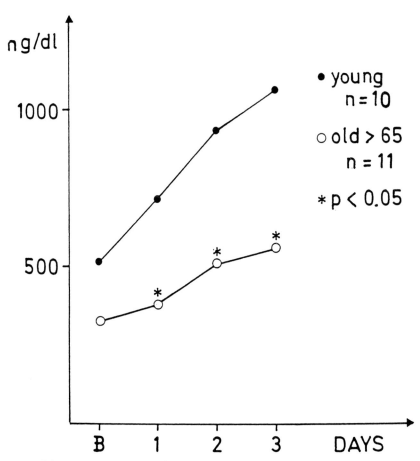

FIGURE 7.3 Testosterone secretion in elderly males in response to an exogenous stimulus. (Human chorionic gonadotrophin [HCG].)

Clinical conclusions

It is apparent that the changes in fertility, sexuality and androgen secretion in old age are highly variable; some elderly men have a very pronounced impairment, while others experience no change at all.

An andropausal syndrome in the strict sense would be exemplified by an elderly male complaining of decreased libido and potency exhibiting slight hypogonadism (gynaecomastia and loss of body hair), fatigue, emotivity and vasomotor disturbances.

Although type I osteoporosis occurs in the male, it is much less prevalent than in the female (1 : 6).

In fact, the incidence of a detectable andropausal syndrome is rather low.

Mastrogiacomo et al.[28] observed decreased testosterone levels and increased LH levels in 26% of aging males. Substitution treatment for the andropausal syndrome has not yet been tested on a large scale. Preliminary communications point towards an important role for the transdermal administration of testosterone/dihydrotestosterone in this field[29,30]. This could alleviate symptoms caused by androgen deficiency. As stated in the introduction, however, the aging process affects not only the endocrine system but also the vascular and neurological systems and these all contribute to a decline in sexual performance with old age.

REFERENCES

1. Beek, C. H. (1950). A Study on extension and distribution of the human body hair. *Dermatologia*, **101**, 317
2. Nutall, F. Q. (1979). Gynecomastia as a physical finding in normal men. *J. Clin. Endocrin. Metab.*, **48**, 338
3. The Bible, *Kings I*, **I**, 1–4
4. Martin, G. E. (1977). Sexual activity in the aging male. In Money J. and Musaph H. (eds.). *Handbook of Sexology*, p. 813– 824. (Amsterdam: Elsevier Science Publishers)
5. Baker, H. W. G., Burger, H. G., de Kretser, D. M. et al. (1976). Changes in the pituitary-testicular system with age. *Clin. Endocr.*, **5**, 349
6. Handelsman, D. J., Staras, S. (1985). Testicular size: the effects of aging, malnutrition and illness. *J. Androl.*, **6**, 144
7. Johnson, L., Petty, C. S., Neaves, W. B. (1984). Influence of age on sperm production and testicular weight in men. *J. Reprod. Fertil.*, **70**, 211
8. Bishop, M. W. H. (1970). Aging and reproduction in the male. *J. Reprod. Fertil.*, (Suppl.) **12**, 65
9. Blum, V. (1936). Das Problem des männlichen Klimakteriums. *Wien. klin. Wschr.*, **2**, 1133
10. Schwartz, D., Mayaux, M. J., Spira, A. et al. (1983). Semen characteristics as a function of age in 833 fertile men. *Fertil. Steril.*, **39**, 530

11. Natoli, A., Riondiono, G., Bracati, A. (1972). Studio della funzione gonadale hormonica e spermatogenetica nel caso della senescenza maschile. *J. Geront.*, **20**, 1103

12. Neaves, W. B., Johnson, L., Porter, J. C. et al. (1984). Leydig cell members, daily sperm production, and serum gonadotrophin levels in aging men. *J. Clin. Endocrin. Metabol.*, **59**, 766

13. Seymour, F. I., Duffy, C., Koerner, A. (1935). A case of authenticated fertility in a man of 94. *J. Amer. Med. Assoc.*, **105**, 1423

14. Anderson, B. A. (1975). Male age and fertility: Results from Ireland prior to 1911. *Population Index*, **41**, 561

15. Vermeulen, A., Rubens, R., Verdonck, L. (1972). Testosterone secretion and metabolism in male senescence. *J. Clin. Endocrin. Metab.*, **34**, 730

16. Pirke, K. M., Doerr, P. (1973). Age related changes and interrelationship between plasma testosterone, oestradiol and testosterone binding globulin in normal adult males. *Acta Endocrin.*, **74**, 792

17. Nieschlag, E., Kley, H. K., Wiegelmann, W. et al. (1973). Lebensalter und endokrine Funktion des Testes der erwachsenen Mannes. *Dtch. med. Wschr.*, **98**, 1281

18. Rubens, R., Dhont, M., Vermeulen, A. (1974). Further studies on Leydig cell function in old age. *J. Clin. Endocrin. Metab.*, **39**, 40

19. Harman, S. M., Tsitouras, P. D. (1980). Reproductive hormones in aging men: I. Measurements of sex steroids, basal luteinizing hormone and Leydig cell response to human chorionic gonadotrophin. *J. Clin. Endocrin. Metab.*, **51**, 35

20. Sparrow, D., Bosse, R., Rowe, J. W. (1980). The influence of age, alcohol consumption and body build in gonadal function in men. *J. Clin. Endocrin. Metab.*, **51**, 508

21. Nieschlag, E., Lammers, U., Freischen, C. W. et al. (1982). Reproductive function in young fathers and grandfathers. *J. Clin. Endocrin. Metab.*, **55**, 676

22. Deslypere, J. P., Vermeulen, A. (1984). Leydig cell function in normal men: effect of age, lifestyle, residence, diet and activity. *J. Clin. Endocrin. Metab.*, **59**, 955

23. Zumoff, B., Strain, G. W., Kream, J. et al. (1982). Age variation of the 24 hours mean plasma concentration of androgens, estrogens and gonadotrophins in normal adult men. *J. Clin. Endocrin. Metab.*, **54**, 538

24. Warner, B. A., Dufau, M. L., Santen, R. J. (1985). Effects of aging and illness on the pituitary testicular axis in men: quantitative as well as qualitative changes in luteinizing hormone. *J. Clin. Endocrin. Metab.*, **60**, 263

25. Deslypere, J. P., Kaufman, J. M., Vermeulen, A. et al. (1987). Influence of age on pulsatile luteinizing hormone release and responsiveness of the gonadotrophins to sex hormone feed-back in men. *J. Clin. Endocrin. Metab.*, **64**, 68

26. Gooren, L. J. G., Van Kessel, H. (1987). The estrogen positive feedback

of LH can be more readily elicited in older men than in young men. (submitted for publication)

27. Harman, S. M., Tsitouras, P. D., Costa, P. T. et al. (1982). Reproductive hormones in aging men: II. Basal pituitary gonadotrophin and gonado-trophin responses to luteinizing hormone-releasing hormone. *J. Clin. Endocrin. Metab.*, **54**, 547

28. Mastrogiacomo, I., Feghari, G., Foresta, C. et al. (1982). Andropause: incidence and pathogenesis. *Arch. Androl.*, **9**, 293

29. Vermeulen, A., Deslypere, J. P. (1985). Long-term transdermal di-hydrotestosterone therapy: effects on pituitary gonadal axis and plasma lipoproteins. *Maturitas*, **7**, 281

30. Findlay, J. C., Place, V. A., Snyder, P. J. (1987). Transdermal delivery of testosterone. *J. Clin. Endocrin. Metab.*, **64**, 266

8

Effects of oestrogens and progestogens on the cardiovascular system in post-menopausal women

Chairman: R. A. Lobo (USA)
Speakers: B. Wren (Australia)
N. Crona (Sweden)
R. Ross (USA)
B. von Schoultz (Sweden)
D. Fraser (UK)

The workshop on the effects of sex steroids on cardiovascular (CV) disease in the climacteric included contributions from B. Wren (Australia), N. Crona (Sweden), R. Ross (United States), B. von Schoultz (Sweden) and D. Fraser (United Kingdom). The effects of oestrogen and progestogens on the incidence of CV disease and on blood pressure, coagulation and lipids were reviewed. In addition, other mechanisms whereby oestrogen influences the CV system were discussed. The following paragraphs represent somewhat of a consensus report on the state of our knowledge in this area.

Prior to the time of menopause coronary heart disease (CHD) is predominantly a male disease with an incidence in men 4–5 times that in women. However, the incidence in women rises sharply at menopause: from 70/100,000 for ages 50–54, to 5040/100,000 for ages 75–79, at which stage the male to female ratio is equal. When the possible causes are analyzed, the most striking of the risk factors involved is seen to be the rise in serum cholesterol. It has been observed that while serum total cholesterol is generally higher in men than in women prior to menopause (223.8 vs 204.8 mg/dl for ages 35–39), this situation is reversed thereafter (229.2 vs 257.1 mg/dl for ages 55–59)[1].

The controversy surrounding the effect of oestrogen on the incidence of CV disease results in large part from data on the potentially delete-rious effects of oral contraceptives on the CV system. Oral contracep-tives containing 50 μg or more of synthetic oestrogen (ethinyl oestra-diol or mestranol) increase the occurrence of conditions such as throm-bosis and hypertension[2,3]. However, these data may not be extrapo-lated to the use of natural oestrogens as prescribed in the menopause. It has been shown that ethinyl oestradiol is at least 200 times more potent than the natural oestrogens in stimulating hepatic globulins[4].

The use of 'natural' oestrogens has been associated with a reduction in the incidence of CV disease in most studies[5-8] (Table 8.1). One smaller study recently suggested that this was not the case[9], but these findings, which are in contradiction to those in many other larger reports, essentially stand alone in this regard. Table 8.1 includes the most convincing cohort studies on the cardioprotective effect of oes-trogen. Although the mechanism whereby 'natural' oestrogen use in the menopause may be cardioprotective has not yet been established, the importance of these observations cannot be ignored in view of the marked reduction in overall mortality associated with even a modest decrease in CHD[10].

It appears that any decrease in the incidence of CV disease is of

Table 8.1 COHORT STUDIES OF OESTROGEN REPLACEMENT THERAPY AND CORONARY HEART DISEASE (CHD)

Investigator/ year	*Study population*	*Description of cohort*	*End- point*	*Relative risk*
Burch et al. 1974[38]	Surgical practice, Nashville, Tenn.	737 hysterectomized women	CHD	0.4
Hammond et al. 1979[6]	Duke Medical Center	610 hypo-oestrogenic inpatients and outpatients	CHD	0.3
Bush et al. 1983[7]	Lipid Research Clinics, USA	2,269 white women	Fatal CHD	0.3
Stampfer et al. 1985[8]	Nurses Health Study, USA	32,317 postmenopausal women	CHD	0.5
Bush et al. 1987[17]	Lipid Research women Clinics, USA	2,270 white	Fatal CHD	0.37

much greater importance than a decrease in any other disease associated with oestrogen therapy[10]. A change in the relative risk (RR) for CV disease from 1 to 0.5 with oestrogen use will result in a reduction in deaths of 5,280/100,000 oestrogen users[11]. It is interesting to compare this with the impact of oestrogen on osteoporosis, where a similar reduction in RR from 1 to 0.5 will result in a reduction of fewer than 500 deaths/100,000 oestrogen users (Table 8.2).

Table 8.2 ESTIMATED CHANGES IN MORTALITY INDUCED BY HIGH AND MODERATE-DOSE OESTROGEN REPLACEMENT THERAPY IN PATIENTS AGED 50 TO 75 YEARS

		High dose		Moderate dose
Condition	*RR*	*Cumulative change in mortality/ 100.000*	*RR*	*Cumulative change in mortality/ 100.000*
Osteoporotic fractures	0.4	−563	0.4	−563
Gallbladder disease	2.0	+3	1.5	+2
Endometrial cancer	7.0	+378*	2.0	+63*
Breast cancer	1.5	+938	1.1	+187
Ischaemic heart disease	0.5	−5250	0.5	−5250
Net change		−4494		−5561
Net % change		33%		−41%

RR = Relative risk
*Case fatality rate for oestrogen-induced endometrial cancer estimated at 0.05.
(From Henderson, B. et al. (1986)[10].)

Because several endogenous risk factors lead to CV disease, the potential impact of sex steroid therapy on each of these needs to be considered. These factors include blood pressure changes, coagulation, lipids and carbohydrate tolerance, as well as the effects of hormonal therapy on life stresses and the quality of life.

Blood pressure

It has generally been assumed that oestrogen increases blood pressure and leads to the development of hypertension. Such assumptions have been extrapolated from data on the use of oral contraceptives and do not reflect the findings relating to the use of hormonal replacement therapy in the climacteric.

The potential danger of inducing blood pressure elevation and hypertension with oestrogen has been unjustifiably magnified. The occurrence of oestrogen-induced hypertension cannot be disputed, but it is seen only rarely, in perhaps 5% of patients[12]. It is important to understand that these cases represent idiosyncratic reactions to oestrogen. The more carefully designed studies on blood pressure responses to post-menopausal oestrogen strongly suggest that both systolic and diastolic blood pressure readings either remain unchanged or are lowered by oestrogen administration, although the decrement may be small[12-14].

Whether the lower level of renin substrate accompanying effective doses of 'natural' oestrogens has any significant clinical effect on blood pressure has not been shown. While an exaggerated activation of the renin-angiotensin system has been implicated in the occurrence of

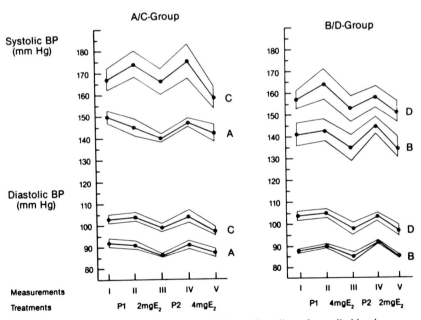

FIGURE 8.1 Effects of micronized oestradiol (E_2) on diastolic and systolic blood pressure in normotensive (Groups A and B) and hypertensive (Groups C and D) women. Shown are mean values ± SEM for blood pressure in supine position (P = placebo).
(From Luotola, H., 1983[14])

hypertension following oestrogen administration, there is no proof that this mechanism is operative. Non oral routes of administration, avoiding direct circulation to the liver, also offer a theoretical clinical advantage. However, no study has directly addressed the issue of hypertension risk with these forms of therapy. There is good evidence to suggest that hypertensive women are good candidates for oestrogen, generally experiencing the same blood pressure response as normotensive women[12,14].

The common assumption that 'natural' oestrogen will frequently induce or aggravate hypertension cannot be supported by current evidence. Oestrogen need not be withheld on the basis of theoretical blood pressure concerns or the presence of hypertension. However, the possibility of a rare idiosyncratic hypertensive response should not be ignored or forgotten.

It appears that in post-menopausal replacement therapy, progestogens play no role in blood pressure changes.

Coagulation factors

While synthetic oestrogens in oral contraceptives clearly affect coagulation factors (in particular, they increase factors VII and X, and decrease antithrombin III), 'natural' oestrogens appear to be devoid of these effects. Furthermore, oestrogen does not appear to increase platelet-derived thromboxane and may increase prostacyclin (as reflected in levels of 6-keto $PGF_1\alpha$). Figure 8.2 depicts data from a double-blind, crossover study[15], where oestrone sulphate and placebo did not affect various clotting parameters, whereas ethinyl oestradiol did. Similar data have also been published regarding the use of conjugated oestrogens[16]. These data suggest that 'natural' oestrogen replacement therapy does not entail a thrombosis risk for post-menopausal women.

The less specific data that are available on progestogens would suggest that they are devoid of independent effects on coagulation factors.

Lipoproteins

The most widely held view regarding the mechanism whereby oestrogens are cardioprotective is that oestrogen favourably affects

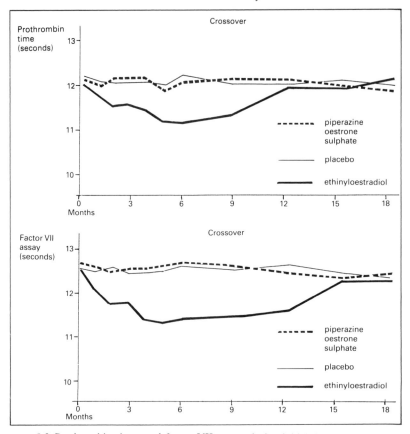

FIGURE 8.2 Prothrombin times and factor VII assays during initial 6-month comparative trial of piperazine oestrone sulphate (3 mg/day), placebo and ethinyl oestradiol (30 μg/day) and during the following 12 months after crossover to piperazine oestrone sulphate (3 mg/day): mean values (± SD with range of 1.4% to 4.2% of mean values)

lipoprotein fractions. There is irrefutable evidence that oral oestrogen use increases high-density-lipoprotein cholesterol (HDL-C) and lowers low-density-lipoprotein cholesterol (LDL-C)[17–19], these being effects that are known to be negatively correlated with cardiovascular risk. Further refinement of these observations has come about with measurements of specific subfractions such as HDL_2C and apoproteins of HDL-C (APO A_1 and A_2), as well as intermediate-density lipoprotein (IDL) and apoprotein B_{100}[20,21].

Oestrogen appears to exert a dose-related effect on HDL-C. Higher doses are more stimulating, as are the effects of synthetic over 'natural' oestrogens. This is primarily thought to be mediated via a decrease in hepatic lipase which helps in the degradation of HDL. These effects appear to be largely mediated via the 'first passage' following oral ingestion and are not usually seen with most types of parenteral oestrogen use.

Recent controversy in this area has revolved around the relative importance of increases in HDL-C (particularly HDL-2b) and APO A_1. This is of relevance to the use of parenteral oestrogens which, because of the lack of a first-passage effect, have an insignificant influence in most studies on HDL-cholesterol. There is evidence, however, that LDL-C levels decrease with time[22] and a growing number of investigators now suggest that the lowering of LDL-C may be more important than the rises in HDL-C observed with oral oestrogens.

While the addition of progestogens to oestrogen therapy is important to prevent endometrial disease[23], progestogens lower HDL-C and in some instances also induce a rise in LDL-C[24]. In recent years, it has been realized that lower doses of progestogens may be sufficient to negate the adverse effect of oestrogen on the endometrium if administered for a sufficient number of days[25,26]. While 19-nor-progestogens appear to be most potent in adversely affecting lipoprotein moieties, even medroxyprogesterone acetate (MPA 10 mg/day) would seem to

Table 8.3 ADJUSTED* PERCENTAGE CHANGE IN LIPIDS AND LIPOPROTEINS BY TYPE OF CONJUGATED OESTROGEN

Type of Oestrogen	Number of Studies	*Change in*			
		Total Chol-esterol	*HDL Chol-esterol*	*LDL Chol-esterol*	*Trigly-cerides*
Equine oestrogens	10	−9%	+10%	− 6%	+20%
Oestradiol valerate	7	−4%	+15%	−16%	+4%
Oestradiol succinate	2	0.0%	+12%	0.0%	+2%
Piperazine oestrone sulphate	4	−6%	+8%	−11%	+7%

*Adjusted for sample size and duration of study.
(From Bush, T. L. et al. (1987)[17])

be detrimental, whereas natural progesterone does not apparently have this property[27]. Recent data suggest that lower doses of MPA (2.5–5 mg) or norethisterone (NET) (1 mg)[28] may not adversely affect lipoproteins or attenuate the beneficial effects of oestrogen use.

Carbohydrate metabolism

There is no evidence that hormonal replacement in post-menopausal women is associated with a deterioration in carbohydrate tolerance. While 19-nor-progestogens contained in oral contraceptives may be implicated in glucose intolerance in women, 'natural' oestrogen use in post-menopausal women is devoid of such an effect. Solid evidence exists to suggest the opposite, namely that oestrogen may improve carbohydrate tolerance by enhancing the action of insulin[29]. Women with diabetes mellitus should not be excluded from receiving hormonal replacement therapy. However, it would be prudent to avoid high doses of 19-nor-progestogens in all post-menopausal women because of such potential adverse affects on carbohydrates as well as on lipoproteins, as discussed above.

Hormonal replacement and quality of life issues

While there are no hard data to confirm the notion that alleviation of life stresses is associated with a reduction in CV risk, conventional wisdom would support this view. Thus, since the cardioprotective mechanisms of oestrogen replacement remain unaltered, it would seem appropriate to examine other facets of the risk-benefit equation. There is no question that oestrogen has a 'mental tonic' effect in post-menopausal women. Significant decreases in anxiety, depression and insomnia, and a generally improved sense of well-being are induced[30]. While these changes may be due largely to the improvement in vasomotor symptoms, data presented at the Congress[31] would suggest that there is an improvement in psychological mood in even asymptomatic women. It therefore appears valid to acknowledge that oestrogen improves the quality of life in post-menopausal women. Some data exist, however, which would suggest that certain progestogens may adversely affect oestrogen's mental tonic effect in susceptible women. Clearly, more information on these issues is needed.

Mechanisms for the cardioprotective effect of oestrogen

While many investigators favour the lipid hypothesis to explain the 50% reduction in CV disease achieved with oestrogen replacement therapy, other oestrogen effects should also be considered. Data presented at the Congress suggest an important direct oestrogen action on arterial vessels. Specific oestradiol receptors, as well as hydroxysteroid dehydrogenase enzyme systems, have been identified in arterial walls. These data suggest a possible direct action by and metabolism of oestrogen in arterial walls. Certain oestrogens have been shown to lower blood pressure[12] as well as to alter blood flow[32-34].

Another important oestrogen mechanism may be stimulation of alterations in prostanoid production. An increase has been observed in the prostacyclin (PGI_2)/thromboxane balance during oestrogen administration[35,36]. While a dose-response increase in PGI_2 has been seen with oestrogen, no changes in thromboxane have been reported. These data are reassuring in regard to platelet-induced proaggregatory effects, and encouraging as far as the vasodilatory function of PGI_2 is concerned.

Oestrogen may stimulate the release of peptides, which are important for vasodilation[37]. Levels of immunoreactive calcitonin gene-related peptide (CGRP) increase in pregnancy and this is one of the most potent naturally-occurring vasodilators known in man. The sex steroid modulation of CGRP may be of importance in post-menopausal women. Thus, it is conceivable that the cardioprotective effect afforded by oestrogen is mediated via a combination of factors which require further elucidation. Only a few of the mechanisms have been covered here. Absolute reliance on the changes in lipoprotein moieties induced by oestrogen may result in other important cardioprotective mechanisms being underestimated.

The use of progestogens in hysterectomized women

It appears that progestogens are extremely important in preventing endometrial disease in women with a uterus. However, there is potential for harm if certain progestogens are used in large doses. These may have adverse effects on lipoproteins, carbohydrate tolerance and mood. In addition, there is growing evidence that the beneficial effect of oestrogen on blood flow, particularly as mediated via the prostanoids, may be inhibited by progestogens, including progesterone. Such data lend credence to the notion that caution is necessary in prescribing progestogens when they may not be necessary, as, for example, in hysterectomized women.

In a vote on this controversial issue, four of the panelists at the Congress were opposed to the use of any progestogen in hysterectomized women, and two were in favour. The principal argument in support of the use of progestogens in hysterectomized women is based on their theoretical protective effect against breast cancer. While this was another controversial issue on which the panelists could not reach a consensus, it was the overall view of the majority of participants and of this Chairperson that there is insufficient evidence to suggest that progestogens have a breast cancer protective effect.

In conclusion, it appears that although there is controversy regarding the effects of oestrogens and progestogens on certain health-related parameters, oestrogen replacement therapy is clearly cardioprotective. Cardioprotection emerges as one of the predominant reasons for prescribing oestrogen to post-menopausal women. One of the major challenges for the remainder of the decade will be to seek to understand and elucidate the mechanisms whereby oestrogen exerts its cardioprotective effect.

REFERENCES

1. Gordon, T., Shurtieff, D. (1973). Means at each examination and interexamination variation of specified characteristics: Framingham Study, Exam 1 to Exam 10. *The Framingham Study: An Epidemiological Investigation of Cardiovascular Disease.* Section 29. (Washington DC: DHEW Publ. No [NIH] 74–478, US Govt. Printing Office)
2. Royal College of General Practitioners (1974). *Oral Contraceptives and Health.* (New York: Pitman Publishing)
3. Royal College of General Practitioners, Oral Contraceptive Study (1978). Oral contraceptives, venous thrombosis and varicose veins. *J. Coll. Gen. Pract.,* **28**, 393
4. Mashchak, C. A., Lobo, R. A., Dozono-Takano, R. et al. (1982). Comparison of pharmacodynamic properties of various estrogen formulations. *Am. J. Obstet. Gynecol.,* **144**, 511
5. Ross, R. K., Paganini-Hill, A., Mack, T. N. et al. (1981). Menopausal estrogen therapy and protection from death from ischemic heart disease. *Lancet,* **1**, 858
6. Hammond, C. B., Jelovsek, F. R., Lee, K. L. et al. (1979). Effects of long-term estrogen replacement therapy. I. Metabolic effects. *Am. J. Obstet. Gynecol.,* **133**, 525

7. Bush, T. L., Cowan, L. D., Barrett-Connor, E. et al. (1983). Estrogen use and all-cause mortality. *J. Am. Med. Assoc.*, **249**, 903

8. Stampfer, M. J., Willett, W. C., Colditz, J. A. et al. (1985). A prospective study of postmenopausal estrogen therapy and coronary heart disease. *N. Eng. J. Med.*, **313**, 1044

9. Wilson, P. W. F., Garrison, R. J., Custelli, W. P. (1985). Postmenopausal estrogen use, cigarette smoking and cardiovascular morbidity in women over 59. *N. Eng. J. Med.*, **313**, 1038

10. Henderson, B. E., Ross, R., Paganini-Hill, A. (1986). Estrogen use and cardiovascular disease. *Am. J. Obstet. Gynecol.*, **154**, 1181

11. Ross, R. K., Paganini-Hill, A., Mack, T. M. et al. (1987). Estrogen use and cardiovascular disease. In Mishell D. R. Jr. (ed.). *Menopause: Physiology and Pharmacology*, pp. 209–223. (Chicago/London: Year Book Medical Publishers, Inc.)

12. Mashchak, C. and Lobo, R. A. (1985). Estrogen replacement therapy and hypertension. *J. Reprod. Med.*, **30**, 805

13. Lind, T., Cameron, E. C., Hunter, W. M. et al. (1979). A prospective, controlled trial of six forms of hormone replacement therapy given to postmenopausal women. *Br. J. Obstet. Gynaecol.* (Suppl.) 3, **86**, 1

14. Luotola, H. (1983). Blood pressure and hemodynamics in postmenopausal women during estradiol-17 substitution. *Ann. Clin. Res.* (Suppl.) 38, **15**, 9

15. Aylward, M., Maddock, J., Rees, P. L. (1976). Natural oestrogen replacement therapy and blood clotting. *Br. Med. J.*, **1**, 220

16. Notelovitz, M., Kitchens, C., Ware, M. et al. (1983). Combination estrogen and progestogen replacement therapy does not adversely affect coagulation. *Obstet. Gynecol.*, **62**, 596

17. Bush, T. L., Barrett-Connor, E., Cowan, L. D. et al (1987). Cardiovascular mortality and non contraceptive use of estrogen in women: results from the Lipid Research Clinic's Program Follow-up Study. *Circulation*, **75**, 1102

18. Wahl, P., Walden, C., Knopp, R. et al. (1982). Effect of estrogen/progestin potency on lipid/lipoprotein cholesterol. *N. Engl. J. Med.*, **208**, 862

19. Barnes, R. B., Roy, S., Lobo, R. A. (1985). Comparison of lipid and androgen levels after conjugated estrogen or depo-medroxyprogesterone acetate treatment in menopausal women. *Obstet. Gynecol.*, **66**, 216

20. Tikkanen, M. J., Nikkila, E. A., Kuuai, T. et al. (1981). Different effects of two progestins on plasma high density lipoprotein (HDL_2) and post-heparin plasma hepatic lipase activity. *Atherosclerosis*, **40**, 365

21. Ottoson, U. P., Johansson, B. G., Von Schoultz, B. (1985). Subfractions of high-density lipoprotein cholesterol during estrogen replacement therapy. A comparison between progestogens and natural progesterone. *Am. J. Obstet. Gynecol.*, **151**, 746

22. Jensen, J., Riis, B. J., Strom, V. et al. (1987). Long term effects of percutaneous estrogens and oral progesterone on serum lipoproteins in postmenopausal women. *Am. J. Obstet. Gynecol.*, **156**, 86

23. Whitehead, M. I., Siddle, N., Lane, G. et al. (1987). The pharmacology of

progestogens. In Mishell, D. R. Jr. (ed.). *Menopause: Physiology and Pharmacology*, pp. 317–334. (Chicago/London: Year Book Medical Publishers, Inc.)

24. Silfverstolpe, G., Gustafson, A., Samsioe, G. et al. (1986). Lipid metabolic studies in oophorectomized women: effects on serum lipids and lipoproteins following different doses of combined postmenopausal replacement therapy. *Br. J. Obstet. Gynecol.*, **93**, 613

25. Nachtigall, L. E., Nachtigall, R. H., Nachtigall, R. D. et al. (1979). Estrogen replacement therapy. I. A 10-year prospective study in the relationship to osteoporosis. *Obstet. Gynecol.*, **53**, 277

26. Riis, B. J., Nilas, L., Christiansen, C. et al. (1984). Effect of oestrogen: progestogen treatment on bone turnover in early postmenopausal women. *Maturitas*, **6**, 169

27. Ottoson, U. P., Johansson, B. G., Von Schoultz, B. (1985). Subfractions of high-density lipoprotein cholesterol during estrogen replacement therapy. A comparison between progestogens and natural progesterone. *Am. J. Obstet. Gynecol.*, **151**, 746

28. Jensen, J., Nilas, L., Christiansen, C. (1986). Cyclic changes in serum cholesterol and lipoproteins following different doses of combined postmenopausal replacement therapy. *Br. J. Obstet. Gynecol.*, **93**, 613

29. Spellacy, W. N. (1987). Menopause, estrogen treatment and carbohydrate metabolism. In Mishell, D. R. Jr. (ed.). *Menopause: Physiology and Pharmacology*, pp. 253–260. (Chicago/London: Year Book Medical Publishers, Inc.)

30. Dennerstein, L. (1987). Psychologic changes. In Mishell, D. R. Jr. (ed.). *Menopause: Physiology and Pharmacology*, pp. 115–127. (Chicago/London: Yearbook Medical Publishers, Inc.)

31. Lobo, R. A., Cristo, M., Crary, W. (1987). Effects of estrogens on psychological function in asymptomatic postmenopausal women. In *Abstracts Fifth International Congress on the Menopause* (Sorrento, Italy), abstract nr. 66

32. Rosenfeld, C., Morris, F. N., Battaglia, F. C. et al. (1976). Effect of estradiol 17α on blood flow to reproductive and nonreproductive tissues in pregnant ewes. *Am. J. Obstet. Gynecol.*, **124**, 618

33. Sarrel, P. M. (1987). Measurement of cutaneous blood flow before and after ovarian hormone replacement therapy in postmenopausal women. In *Abstracts Fifth International Congress on the Menopause* (Sorrento, Italy), abstract nr. 135

34. Semmens, J., Tsai, C. C., Semmens, E. C. et al. (1984). Changes in vaginal physiology during the menopause and the effect in exogenous estrogen therapy. *Maturitas*, **6**, 179

35. Silfverstolpe, G., Enk, L., Kallfelt, B. et al. (1984). Effects of exogenous estrogen on the prostacyclin/thromboxane balance in oophorectomized women. *Maturitas*, **6**, 184

36. Makila, U. M., Wahlberg, L., Viinikka, L. et al. (1982). Regulation of prostacyclin and thromboxane production by human umbilical vessels: the

effect of estradiol in superfusion model. *Prostag. Leukotrienes Med.,* **8**, 115

37. Whitehead, M., Fraser, D. (1987). Controversies concerning the safety of estrogen replacement therapy. *Am. J. Obstet. Gynecol.,* **156**, 1313
38. Burch, J. C., Byrd, B. F., Vaughn, W. K. (1974). The effects of long-term estrogen on hysterectomized women. *Am. J. Obstet. Gynecol.,* **118**, 778

9

Neuroendocrine treatment of the menopause

Chairman: A. Genazzani (Italy)
Co-chair: G. Ginsburg (UK)
Speakers: F. Petraglia (Italy)
J. Ginsburg (UK)
G. Melis (Italy)

Many recent reports indicate that neuroactive drugs may be useful in the treatment of menopausal symptoms. There are two major reasons for this new therapeutic perspective: firstly, improved knowledge of the underlying pathophysiology and, secondly, the opportunity such drugs offer to avoid the possible risks associated with oestrogen replacement therapy (endometrial and breast cancer, hypertension).

Three neural pathways have accordingly been investigated, viz endogenous opioid peptides (EOPs), the adrenergic/noradrenergic system and the dopaminergic system.

Petraglia presented the results that have been obtained in the Department of Obstetrics and Gynaecology at the University of Modena using naloxone in the treatment of menopausal hot flushes. Naloxone is an opiate-receptor antagonist. It is a safe drug with a short half-life that is effective in relieving the frequency of flushes in menopausal women. The rationale for its use is that opioid peptides (endorphins, enkephalins, dynorphins) induce hot flushes when injected into healthy subjects. Anatomical and biochemical findings indicate that EOPs play an important role in the control of the thermoregulatory centre in the hypothalamus. The decrease in the number of hot flushes that results from blocking the opiate receptors with naloxone may thus be explained by its antagonism to the endogenous substances which are the central cause.

A link between hot flushes and the neuroendocrinology of the hypothalamic control of gonadotrophin-releasing hormone (GnRH) has been previously suggested. It was considered that the correlation between hot flushes and plasma surges of luteinizing hormone (LH) levels might be a fundamental factor in the occurrence of flushing. Petraglia emphasized the basic and clinical data demonstrating the role of EOPs in the regulation of LH secretion. Several reports indicate that EOPs tonically inhibit the secretion of LH, acting at the hypothalamic level. The blockade of opiate receptors is accompanied by an increase in plasma LH. Naloxone sharply increases LH levels in animals and humans. Interestingly, this neuroendocrine effect is sensitive to the circulating levels of gonadal steroids. In castrated subjects and in post-menopausal women, naloxone does not modify LH levels. However, following steroid replacement treatment, the modulation of LH by EOPs is restored, as is shown by the significant increase in plasma LH after naloxone administration.

This functional correlation is also associated with a significant change in EOP concentrations in the hypothalamus. The menopause might consequently represent a critical period in life characterized by failure of the activity of the opioid system. The changes involved may be responsible for the alterations in the neuroendocrine, behavioural and functional activities typical of this period of life. The most intriguing problem is the difficulty of manipulating the opiatergic system. It is well-known that opiate receptors quickly develop tolerance, leading to a need for very high therapeutic doses. Moreover, the half-life of naloxone is too short and necessitates continuous infusion to maintain adequate concentrations.

However, taking all factors into consideration, we may assume that drugs acting on opiate receptors could represent an alternative approach in the treatment of menopausal hot flushes.

Ginsburg emphasized that in assessing the potential use and effectiveness of an adrenergic agonist such as clonidine for treating vasomotor climacteric symptoms, it was essential to define the nature of the response under treatment. Many workers had used cutaneous temperature as a measure of the menopausal hot flush and of the effects of treatment on climacteric symptoms. However, as Ginsburg explained, cutaneous temperature represents the difference between heat lost to the environment and that conveyed to the skin by the blood. It is also essential for the body to be dry, since evaporation of water from moist skin will influence the measurements and introduce a possible source of error. This is extremely important when using skin temperature measurements to indicate cutaneous blood flow during the occurrence of menopausal hot flushes, which is itself associated with sweating.

At higher rates of flow, skin temperature is an insensitive and unreliable index of local circulation.

Using venous occlusion plethysmography, which enables frequent quantitative measurements of peripheral blood flow to be made (as often as six times a minute), Ginsburg had shown that there was a marked and rapid increase in hand blood flow which persisted for several minutes after the flush sensations had subsided. There was a simultaneous but smaller rise in forearm flow which fell to basal levels before that in the hand, as well as a significant increase in pulse rate, which also fell to basal levels while hand blood flow was still elevated. There was no change in mean blood pressure during a menopausal hot flush.

A similar response can be demonstrated in the male experiencing debilitating attacks of flushing associated with sweating after bilateral orchidectomy.

Menopausal flushes have often been linked to emotional blushing because of the similar distribution of the cutaneous colour change. However, the pattern of vascular response during an emotional blush is quite different from that observed in menopausal women or in males after orchidectomy. During an emotional blush, there is an increase in forearm blood flow, but no change in hand flow or any rise in blood pressure.

Using strain-gauge plethysmography to evaluate the relative changes in blood flow in skin and muscle vessels during the menopausal flush and emotional blush, Ginsburg was further able to demonstrate that in the former the essential change in flow was in the arterioles of the skin, whereas in the latter a rise in muscle flow was mainly responsible for the increase in forearm flow. In fact, vascular-response pattern during the emotional blush resembled that evoked during stress, whereas the response during menopausal flushing resembled that caused by indirect heating.

Ginsburg also analyzed the standard hypothesis advanced to explain the menopausal hot flush, for which, as she demonstrated, there is no evidence.

In addition, she identified possible sites at which an alpha-agonist might act and consequently alleviate or prevent menopausal flushing. By means of quantitative techniques for measuring peripheral blood flow, Ginsburg and her team had shown that after treatment with clonidine, an alpha-agonist used in the treatment of migraine and the prevention of menopausal hot flushes, dilator responses to vasoactive agents such as adrenaline and angiotensin were reduced. This provided a rationale for the use of clonidine in menopausal flushing and also illustrated a method for testing substances used to treat such flushing. The third speaker, *Melis*, presented the results of his group's investigations to assess the clinical efficacy of bromocriptine as a dopamine-receptor agonist in the control of vasomotor symptoms. Bromocriptine was shown to be capable of reducing both the frequency and the intensity of post-menopausal hot flushes. It was therefore hypothesized that a decrease in the activity of the endogenous dopaminergic system could represent the cause of thermoregulatory instability in post-menopausal women. On the other hand, the antidopaminergic compound veralipride was also shown to be very effective in treating hot flushes. In a cross-over study, both bromocriptine and veralipride showed the same clinical efficacy in the control of hot flushes.

A multicentre clinical trial was consequently performed with a view to defining more clearly the role played by the dopaminergic system in the pathogenesis of hot flushes. Seventy-five post-menopausal women were randomly allocated to five treatment groups. Two groups were treated with a dopaminergic drug (either bromocriptine or liposom), two with an antidopaminergic drug (either veralipride or domperidone) and the remaining group with placebo. Liposom was selected for its ability to act by stimulating endogenous dopamine secretion. Domperidone was selected as a specific dopamine-receptor blocking agent with no central effects, since it does not cross the blood-brain barrier. All four drugs proved to be more effective than placebo in alleviating vasomotor symptoms. These data confirmed that either direct (bromocriptine) or indirect (liposom) dopaminergic stimulation may control hot flushes. In addition, the ability of domperidone to relieve vasomotor symptoms suggested that the clinical efficacy of antidopaminergic drugs such as veralipride and domperidone in controlling hot flushes is independent of their central activity and is probably due to peripheral changes induced by their administration, such as hyperprolactinaemia.

Melis also emphasized the possible role of the endogenous opioid system in the pathogenesis of post-menopausal hot flushes.

The hypothesis that the antidopaminergic drug, veralipride, may control vasomotor symptoms by interfering with the endogenous opioid system was indirectly tested on a group of post-menopausal women by evaluating LH response to naloxone infusion before and after 30 days of veralipride administration (200 mg/day). Before the veralipride treatment, LH plasma levels did not vary significantly during naloxone infusion, whereas they rose significantly afterwards. These data demonstrated that veralipride restores endogenous opioid activity in post-menopausal women and suggested that this action may explain, in part at least, the drug's clinical efficacy in controlling vasomotor symptoms. Since, in previous clinical trials, both veralipride and bromocriptine demonstrated a similar ability to reduce hot flushes, the possibility that bromocriptine might modify endogenous opioid activity was also evaluated in a group of post-menopausal women. LH responses to naloxone infusion before and after 30 days of bromocriptine administration (5 mg/day) was again used as an indirect means of evaluating the effects of this treatment on endogenous opioid activity. LH response to naloxone was absent in untreated post-menopausal women, but was present after bromocriptine administration.

On the basis of the wealth of data provided by the various speakers, it may be concluded that both chronic manipulation of the dopaminergic system and oestrogen administration stimulate the endogenous opioid system in post-menopausal women, and the restoration of endogenous opioidergic tone may represent the mechanism which mediates the clinical efficacy of all these drugs in alleviating vasomotor symptoms. Moreover, since other neuroactive drugs that are effective in treating hot flushes, such as clonidine, also interfere with the endogenous opioid system, it would seem reasonable to suggest that drugs used in the treatment of vasomotor symptoms induce thermoregulatory stability by increasing endogenous opioid activity.

10

Contraception in the pre-menopause

Chairwoman: G. V. UPTON (USA)
Speakers: S. BELISLE (CANADA), E. HIRVONEN (FINLAND), R.
TUIMALA (FINLAND), J. W. W. STUDD, (UK)

The subject of contraception in women aged over 35 presents some
very special challenges to the physician. Many unknown factors play a
role in the normal physiology of women in this age group and many
variables complicate the decision as to which contraceptive approach is
the most appropriate. It is common experience that women in these
years of change have both irregular bleeding (sometimes profuse) and
irregular cycles. To date, there have been no adequate studies on the
requirements of such older women, in whom slow and unpredictable
physiological changes are taking place.

There is a growing awareness that many women aged over 40 require both contraceptive protection and hormonal replacement therapy
for climacteric symptoms. These women are still menstruating and the
risk of pregnancy remains, overshadowed by the increased life-
threatening risk associated with childbirth in this age group. The risk
of mortality due to the use of oral contraceptives is little increased for
the nonsmoking woman in the years beyond 40 as compared with the
years before this critical age. In contrast, women aged over 40 who
smoke are best advised not to use hormonal contraceptives. It is
evident from all the existing data that combination therapy is strongly
advisable if any replacement therapy is to be given. There is a considerable body of evidence which suggests that oestrogen alone may be
insufficient and that progestogen should be added to prevent endometrial hyperplasia, decrease the risk of breast cancer and prevent bone
loss. In the pre-menopausal woman, such therapy should also provide
contraceptive protection.

In attempting to select a contraceptive product it is essential to have
some knowledge of the sensitivity of the pituitary-ovarian axis. No

study has been conducted to date that has adequately defined the parameters concerned in even the normal woman aged over 40. Will these women need more or less hormone to inhibit ovulation? What type of oestrogen should be used – natural or synthetic? Most important of all, how much oestrogen should be used? As regards the progestogen, the question that arises is how much will be necessary to protect against endometrial carcinoma. What dose of progestogen will preclude unwanted metabolic changes? In addition, the fear of adverse cardiovascular effects is ever-present and life-styles seem to play a significant role.

The widespread use of tubal ligation to circumvent the use of hormones in the 35+ woman ignores her inevitable hormonal needs at a later stage in her life.

Where there are contraindications to oestrogen therapy, the availability of other forms of contraception becomes an important consideration. IUDs are not available in the United States. Condoms, diaphragms, sponges and cervical caps do remain as alternatives, but none will suffice as replacement therapy. A need consequently exists for research aimed at discovering non-steroidal therapy that could replace the action of the missing hormones – a challenge that will be difficult to meet.

There were four speakers at this workshop: S. Belisle is studying the climacteric by using C57B1 mice to define the normal aging process, E. Hirvonen and R. Tuimala have each studied new combination products containing oestradiol valerate (E_2V) and ethinyl oestradiol (EE) respectively in human trials and, finally, J. Studd has investigated a contraceptive approach using a different delivery system, viz subcutaneous implantation, for the oestradiol (E_2) component.

1. Kinetics of E_2 receptors throughout the aging of the reproductive systems in C57B1 mice (S. Belisle)

The working hypothesis is that at menopause a change occurs in the set point at which circulating steroids from various sources will inappropriately block or stimulate the secretion of luteinizing hormone releasing hormone (LHRH), which in turn controls the pituitary secretion of gonadotrophins, i.e. follicle-stimulating hormone (FSH) and luteinizing hormone (LH) (Figure 10.1).

Menopause seems to occur as a result of two main factors:

1) Aging of extragonadal oestrogen target sites, of which the brain is

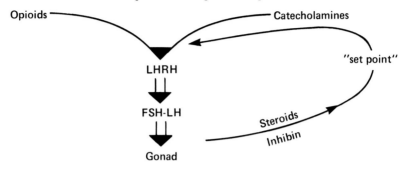

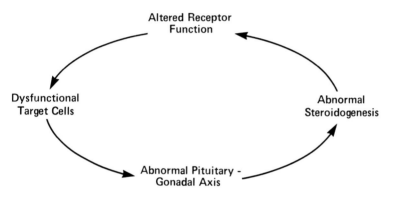

FIGURE 10.1 Working hypothesis of the physiological hormonal changes that mark the menopause.

the most important. Thus, aging of the pituitary, uterus or any other oestrogen target organs, such as the blood vessels or skin, will result clinically in altered cyclicity, delayed feedback and dysfunctional uterine bleeding, as well as increased pregnancy loss.

2) Follicular atresia which develops subsequently and then results in the onset of ovarian acyclicity – the so-called clinical menopause.

Laboratory studies: Biochemical characterization of oestrogen receptors (ER) in the brain and the uterus of C57B1 mice showed a decrease in concentration relative to age. Kinetic studies showed decreased activation of ER early in middle age superimposed on a decreased capacity for the nuclei to bind activated ER after the onset of ovarian acyclicity.

These endocrine changes were present at both tissue sites, appeared to be gonadal-independent but age-dependent, and were paralleled by decreased induction of E_2-specific biological end points, viz G6PDH activity and synthesis of progesterone receptors. Current studies to dissociate the receptor from the nuclear components of these dysfunctional ER complexes have shown a reduction in the dissociation kinetics of ER, as well as an enhanced inhibition of ER activation in uterine cytosols in both middle and old age.

Conclusions: The results suggest the presence of dysfunctional ER in both the brain and uterus of mice as early as middle age and prior to the onset of ovarian acyclicity. These data reflect a physiological impact on both the increased menstrual dysfunction and the higher reproductive losses observed in this age group.

2. Oral contraceptives containing oestradiol valerate for premenopausal women (E. Hirvonen)

Two new formulations, A and B (Figure 10.2), containing oestradiol valerate (E_2V) combined with either cyproterone acetate (A) or norethisterone (B) were studied.

Fifty healthy ovulating women aged between 35 and 47 (mean age 39) received either Formulation A ($n = 26$) or Formulation B ($n = 24$). The subjects were assigned to the groups in a double-blind, random fashion. No pregnancies occurred during administration of either formulation. In Group A, 21 out of 26 (81%) and in Group B 16 out of 24 (67%) completed the first year. The mid-cycle serum FSH and LH peaks were suppressed, while there were no differences in the serum oestradiol values between pretreatment and treatment cycles. Serum progesterone values indicated that only one ovulatory cycle occurred during the first year in Group A, whereas 11 occurred in Group B. Ultrasonic studies revealed follicular growth during treatment in both groups, most follicles becoming atretic or persistent without ovulation.

No significant changes were observed in twelve coagulation factors studied in 16 women in Group A. Serum total cholesterol decreased by about 10% ($p < 0.001$) in both groups, while high-density lipoprotein (HDL) cholesterol concentration fell by 12% ($p < 0.001$) in Group B and also demonstrated a tendency to decrease in Group A.

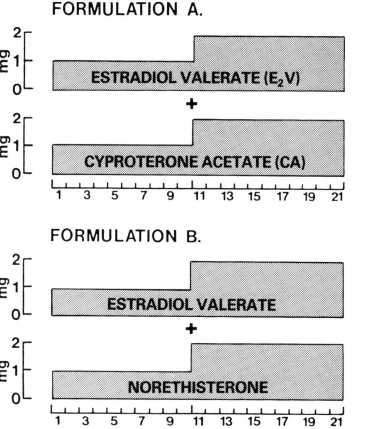

FIGURE 10.2 Formulation A and Formulation B – Two new experimental formulations containing natural oestrogen.

In Group A bleeding became scanter and dysmenorrhoea was eliminated. The incidence of spotting varied between 30 and 40%, but the total number of all bleeding days per cycle decreased.

One woman in Group A and four in Group B discontinued the treatment because of breakthrough bleeding.

It was concluded that natural oestradiol is suitable for use in oral contraceptives and that the oestradiol valerate/cyproterone acetate combination is preferred because it consistently inhibits ovulation, provides tolerable cycle control and does not cause adverse metabolic side effects.

3. Contraception with Mercilon in women aged over 30 (R. Tuimala)

The contraceptive efficacy, cycle control and side effects of a combination of 150 mcg of desogestrel and 20 mcg ethinyl oestradiol (Mercilon) were evaluated. Four hundred and thirty-four (434) women between 30 and 39 years of age participated in an open multicentre study and were followed up through 7,669 cycles. Irregular bleeding occurred in about 25% of the women in the initial months of use but after 12 months only 10% reported irregular bleeding.

No pregnancies occurred, showing that the combination studied was highly effective. Withdrawal bleeding occurred in 87.7% of the women after treatment cycle 1, in 91.5% after cycle 6 and in 94% after cycle 12.

A regular cycle with no irregular bleeding (spotting or breakthrough bleeding) was reported by 74.4% of the subjects after the first cycle, by 85.6% after six cycles and by 91.0% after 12 cycles.

Only minor side effects were noted and at 12 cycles these included nausea 0.4%, headaches 4.9%, nervousness 3.0% and breast tenderness 4.5%. Thereafter the incidence decreased.

A total of 6.9% of the women withdrew from treatment because of these side effects and 6.2% because of irregular bleeding. Adverse effects were seen in two cases, in the form of superficial thrombophlebitis, and the oral contraceptive treatment was stopped in these women.

HDL-cholesterol, % HDL-cholesterol in total cholesterol, sex-hormone binding globulin (SHBG), apolipoprotein A-1, glycosylated proteins and plasma antithrombin III activity were studied in a smaller subgroup of 25 women. Blood samples were taken before treatment and after 1, 3, 6 and 12–15 treatment cycles.

The contraceptive combination had no effect on total cholesterol, glycosylated proteins or antithrombin III activity. During treatment there were small but significant increases in HDL-cholesterol, % HDL-cholesterol in total cholesterol and apolipoprotein A-1, and a substantial increase in SHBG (see Figure 10.3).

It was concluded that a combination of 0.150 mg desogestrel and 0.020 mg ethinyl oestradiol is a safe and highly effective oral contraceptive in women aged 30 or over. Cycle control was good and acceptance excellent. No adverse effects on lipid or carbohydrate metabolism were observed over 12 to 15 treatment cycles.

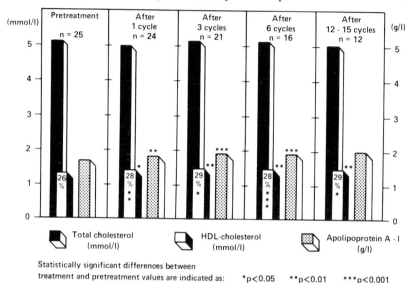

FIGURE 10.3 Mean values of total cholesterol, HDL-cholesterol, %HDL-cholesterol and apolipoprotein A-1. Lipid profiles over 15 months.

4. Use of oestradiol implants for contraception in pre-menopausal women (J. Studd)

Sex hormone implants have been available for almost 50 years, but only a few clinicians administer them regularly. Implants represent a physiological mode of therapy with many metabolic advantages over other routes. Surprisingly, they are largely ignored by physicians. This may well reflect their surgical nature, although the technique of hormone implantation is simple and fast and obviates daily oral medication.

The use of E_2 implants has been extended to pre-menopausal women. The first publication reported on the immediate effects of 100 mg of E_2 and suggested that ovulation can be suppressed by this dose immediately, provided the pellet is inserted early in the cycle[1]. While this may be so in the majority of cases, we found that follicular development continued in almost half the patients studied during the first three cycles after the initial implant, with evidence of follicular rupture and luteinization in a small proportion up to that time (Figure 10.4).

No advantage was gained by using a higher dose of 150 mg E_2. Plasma E_2 levels during the first 6 months of treatment were comparable to those seen in post-menopausal women receiving the same treatment. The potency of this route of therapy is also confirmed by the observations reported in 1954 by Greenblatt et al.[2], who showed that up to 7.5 mg/day of oral equine oestrogens are required to suppress ovarian function, a dose that is 6 to 12 times higher than the standard menopausal replacement dose.

The effects of regular therapy in this age group depend on dosage. With regular 6-monthly implants of 50 mg E_2, the gradual accumulation trend is the same as that seen in post-menopausal women. In our study, 13% of women who had been treated for longer than 3 to 4 years had supraphysiological plasma levels of E_2, but not of oestrone (E_1). Pertinent to this finding is the fact that Greenblatt and his co-workers[1] had earlier shown that the dose of E_2 can be reduced every 6 months to a maintenance level of 25 mg without any loss of contraceptive effect. This regimen avoided any accumulation of plasma E_2 levels, although the same group of investigators subsequently reported that E_2 levels did increase slightly[3].

The hypothesis that the many non-specific changes normally associated with cyclical ovarian activity are the primary aetiological factors in the premenstrual syndrome was tested by suppressing ovulation with subcutaneous E_2 implants. Sixty-eight (68) women with proven premenstrual syndrome were treated under placebo-controlled conditions for up to 10 months in a longitudinal study. Active treatment was combined with cyclical oral norethisterone to produce regular withdrawal periods. Symptoms were monitored by means of daily menstrual distress questionnaires, visual analogue scales, and the 60-item general health questionnaire. Of the 35 women treated with placebo, 33 improved, giving an initial placebo response rate of 94%. The placebo effect gradually waned, but the response to the active combination was maintained for the duration of the study. Analysis of the prospective symptom ratings showed a significant superiority of E_2 implants over placebo after two months for all six symptom clusters in the menstrual distress questionnaire. Changes seen in the retrospective assessments were less significant, but the trend was the same (Figure 10.5).

Treatment with E_2 implants and cyclical progestogen was well tolerated and appears to be both rational and effective for severe cases of the premenstrual syndrome.

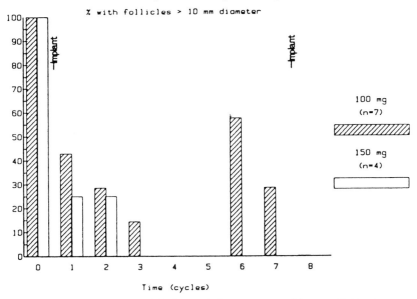

FIGURE 10.4 Follicular growth before and after treatment with oestradiol implants.

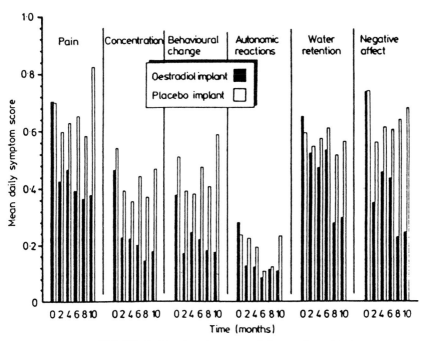

FIGURE 10.5 Effect of treatment on mean daily symptom scores.

REFERENCES

1. Greenblatt, R. B., Asch, R. H., Mahesh, V. B. et al. (1977). Implication of pure crystalline pellets of estradiol for conception control. *Am. J. Obstet. Gynecol.*, **127**, 520
2. Greenblatt, R. B., Hammond, D. O. and Clark, S. L. (1954). Membranous dysmenorrhea: studies in etiology and treatment. *Am. J. Obstet. Gynecol.*, **68**, 835
3. Asch, R. H., Greenblatt, R. B. and Mahesh, V. B. (1978). Pure crystalline estradiol pellet implantation for contraception. *Int. J. Fertil.*, **23**, 100

11

Post-menopausal bone loss and osteoporosis

Chairman: J. C. Stevenson (UK)
Co-chair: G. F. Mazzuoli (Italy)
　　Speakers: R. Lindsay (USA), L. J. Melton III (USA), H. K.
Genant (USA), C. Christiansen (Denmark), C. Gennari (Italy)

Introduction

Over the past decade there has been growing awareness of the size and extent of the post-menopausal oesteoporosis problem[1]. This is now one of the major public health problems of the western world, involving considerable morbidity, mortality and cost. Our insight into the pathogenesis of the condition is now allowing us to initiate rational and effective treatment, particularly in terms of prevention. Newly developed techniques for accurate and precise bone density measurements are enabling us to assess the skeleton at the clinically relevant sites[2] and to detect changes at an early stage. The workshop speakers covered a number of different topics relating to post-menopausal osteoporosis and its development.

Aetiology of osteoporosis (R. Lindsay)

Lindsay began by comparing osteoporosis with hypertension. Hypertension is diagnosed by the detection of elevated blood pressure and treatment is directed at reversing or limiting rises in blood pressure with the ultimate aim of preventing cerebrovascular accident. Osteoporosis is now diagnosed by the detection of decreased bone mass and treatment is directed at reversing or limiting loss of bone with the ultimate aim of preventing fracture. The importance of preventing osteoporosis was emphasized with scanning electron micrographs showing osteoporotic trabecular bone. The loss of trabeculae

125

means the destruction of the anatomical template on which new bone can be built. Hence, osteoporosis eventually becomes irreversible.

Osteoporosis is aetiologically heterogeneous; various factors have an eventual influence on peak adult bone mass and subsequent bone loss (Table 11.1). There is realistically little chance of influencing the factors affecting peak bone mass, these being mainly genetic factors and perhaps nutritional. More important is the menopause which, by accelerating bone turnover (and resorption more than formation), results in fairly rapid loss of bone for up to 8–10 years[3].

Table 11.1 SOME KNOWN AND PUTATIVE POSITIVE AND NEGATIVE RISK FACTORS FOR OSTEOPOROSIS

1. Ovarian function

2. Race

3. Others   – Genetic   e.g. family history
                                 height

             – Life style   e.g. exercise
                                 weight
                                 smoking
                                 parity
                                 oral contraceptive use

           – Nutritional e.g. alcohol
                                 calcium
                                 caffeine

           – Pre-existing skeletal disease

The greater importance of loss of ovarian function as compared with aging was emphasized by a study from the Mayo Clinic[4]. One group comprised women of roughly 50 years of age who had undergone bilateral ovariectomy some 20 years previously, and a second group was made up of women aged roughly 70 who had undergone a spontaneous menopause some 20 years previously. Despite the difference of 20 years in chronological age, no difference in bone density between the groups was apparent.

The importance of calcium intake is no longer convincing. Epidemiological data concerning osteoporosis and calcium are conflicting[5,6] and probably reflect racial rather than dietary calcium differences. Previous estimates for calcium requirements have been derived from balance studies[7]. These are inappropriate, however, since the body protects itself from high calcium intake by changes in the regulating hormones. It would thus not be possible for increased calcium intake itself to produce a positive calcium balance in a post-menopausal woman. There is clearly a threshold for necessary dietary calcium intake, but humans are probably well adapted to a relatively low calcium diet.

Epidemiological aspects (L. J. Melton III)

Melton described the bimodal incidence of limb fractures, with the first peak occurring in young males due to trauma and the second in post-menopausal females due to osteoporosis. The pattern of fracture incidence for the distal forearm shows a sharp increase around the time of menopause and a later flattening with increasing age. This contrasts with the pattern of fracture incidence for the proximal femur, which increases gradually after the menopause but rises more sharply thereafter with increasing age. The pattern for vertebral fractures is intermediate[8] (Figure 11.1).

The critical bone density below which fractures could readily occur – the fracture threshold – is 2 to 3 standard deviations below that of young normals. However, although the mean bone density in patients with hip fracture is lower than that in controls, a bone density measurement is insufficient to discriminate between fracture cases and age-matched controls. Nevertheless, bone density measurements have been correlated with fracture incidence. In a study from the Mayo Clinic, it was found that in patients with a bone density greater than 1.0 g/cm^2 the hip fracture incidence was low, being of the order of less than 0.4 per 1,000 patient-years. However, the hip fracture rate increased 20 to 40-fold in patients with a bone density of less than 0.6 g/cm^2. The findings were similar for spine fractures when bone density was compared with fracture prevalence. However, bone density alone is not sufficient to explain all fractures. Certain fractures, particularly those of the distal forearm and proximal femur, generally require the trauma of a fall. Indeed, the increased propensity of the elderly to fall is regarded by some as the major cause of the higher fracture rate in this age group. This concept is not supported by the findings of a study which investigated falls in a nursing home[9]. Out of

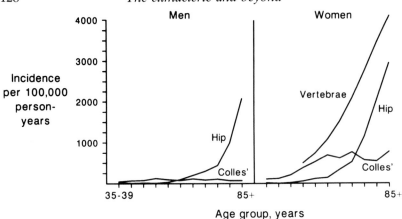

FIGURE 11.1 Incidence rates for the three common osteoporotic fractures (Colles', hip and vertebral) in men and women plotted as function of age at time of fracture. Data are from the community population of Rochester, Minnesota. (Reproduced with permission of authors and *N. Engl. J. Med.*[8])

651 such falls, only 8 resulted in hip fracture. Thus, falls alone are also insufficient to explain all fractures.

If all limb fractures are considered, the excess of the observed over the expected incidence shows that at least 50% are due to osteoporosis. Data on survival following hip fracture reveal an increased mortality, particularly during the first 4 months. The cost of osteoporosis and its attendant fractures is enormous, the current estimates for the USA being over $6 billion annually[10]. At least 15% of all women sustain a hip fracture during their lives. This is similar to the lifetime risk of developing carcinoma of the breast, ovary and uterus combined.

Obviously, many factors affect bone mass, but the combination of low bone mass and trauma results in fracture. Preventive treatment would have a major impact on fracture incidence even if bone loss was only slowed down rather than arrested completely. In the case of hip fracture, a 5-year shift in the incidence curve would result in a reduction of around 50% due to the age of the population at risk (Figure 11.2).

Diagnostic techniques (H. K. Genant)

Genant reviewed the three most commonly used techniques for measuring bone density, namely single photon absorptiometry, dual

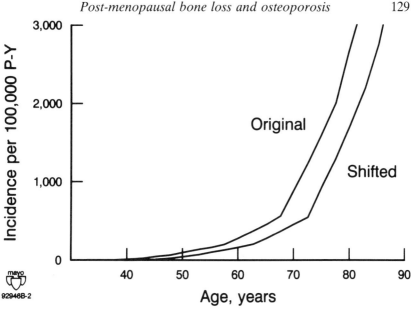

FIGURE 11.2 Age-specific incidence of proximal femur fracture among Rochester, Minnesota, women as originally reported and as it might appear if osteoporosis onset were delayed or progression slowed sufficiently to shift each rate to an age-group 5 years older.

photon absorptiometry and quantitative computed tomography. Single photon absorptiometry measures bone density in the peripheral skeleton and has the advantages of being cheap and easy to perform, with low radiation exposure[11]. It has been shown to be useful for population studies, but is not particularly suitable for osteoporosis screening because of the poor correlation of the results obtained with spine bone density and fractures[12]. Some improvement is gained by measuring ultradistal sites of the forearm which contain relatively larger amounts of trabecular bone[13]. Another approach is to measure the calcaneus, which also contains trabecular bone and is thought to be a good predictor for fracture. However, the density of this bone is particularly affected by body weight and physical activity. It is therefore premature to suggest that mass screening of post-menopausal women with single photon absorptiometry should be adopted.

Dual photon absorptiometry[14,15] has the advantage of measuring bone density at the clinically important sites, i.e. the spine and femoral neck. There is relatively low radiation exposure and it can also be used to measure total body bone mineral, although this remains primarily a research tool. A disadvantage in the elderly is that the measurement includes extravertebral calcification which, in extreme cases, can account for 20–30% of the apparent bone density.

Quantitative computed tomography is able to separate trabecular from cortical bone in the spine[16]. Since trabecular bone is metabolically 8 times more active, the decrement with age is greatest in this site. Precision is good, but accuracy in the elderly can be adversely affected by increased marrow fat[17]. The correlation coefficient for single energy computed tomography with spinal ash weight is 0.96, but the standard error of the estimate is high. However, this error is small when compared with the range of densities that exists between the normal and disease levels, and fairly reliable identification of patients with osteoporosis can be achieved[18].

All methods of bone density measurements have both advantages and disadvantages, some of which are shown in Table 11.2. There is no doubt that region-specific measurements are very important[2,19] and the ability to measure axial bone density is paramount.

Table 11.2 COMPARISON BETWEEN QUANTITATIVE COMPUTED TOMOGRAPHY (QCT), DUAL PHOTON ABSORPTIOMETRY (DPA) AND SINGLE PHOTON ABSORPTIOMETRY (SPA)

Measurement site	QCT spine	DPA spine	SPA mid radius	SPA ultra distal R
Trabecular (%)	100	20–40	5	40–60
Sensitivity	3–4X	2X	1X	1–2X
Precision (%)	1–5	2–4	1–2	1–2
Accuracy (%)	5–15	4–?	5	?
Radiation (MREM)	100–500	10–20	10	15
Time (min)	10	30	10	15
Cost ($)	100–200	100–150	50–125	50–125

Prevention of bone loss (C. Christiansen)

Christiansen reviewed studies on prevention of post-menopausal bone loss conducted in his department with co-workers over the past 10 years. Using mainly single and to a lesser extent dual photon absorptiometry they have been unable to demonstrate significant loss of bone before the menopause. Large studies of early post-menopausal bone loss have shown that Vitamin D metabolites are totally ineffective, as are small doses of fluoride[20]. A large supplement of calcium had no effect on bone loss at the clinically relevant spine and distal forearm sites, but a minimal slowing of forearm cortical bone loss was observed[21]. Any effects that calcitonin may have in the prevention of bone loss are not as yet known. It is thus obvious that there is currently no alternative to oestrogen and progestogen therapy. Their studies have shown that with such treatment a 10% difference in bone density compared with that in placebo controls is observed after 3 years[22] (Figure 11.3). The optimal dose of oral oestradiol is between 1 and 2 mg daily (Figure 11.4).

Since there is a greater percentage change in biochemical parameters than in bone after the menopause, they have attempted to use such parameters to identify women losing bone at a fast rate. On the basis

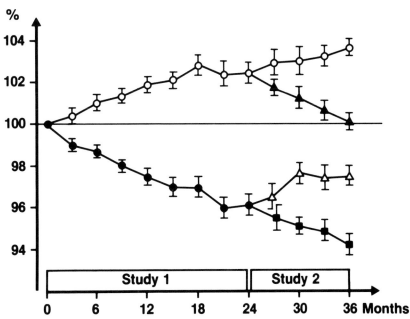

FIGURE 11.3 Bone mineral content during treatment and after withdrawal of hormone. (Reproduced with permission of authors and *Lancet*[22].)

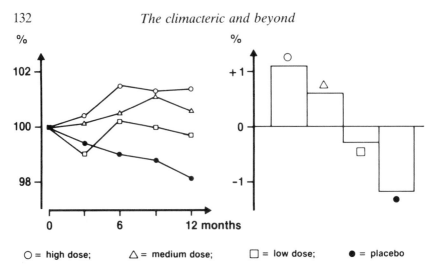

O = high dose;   △ = medium dose;   □ = low dose;   ● = placebo

FIGURE 11.4 Dose-response of bone mineral content (% initial value) to high-dose (4 mg), medium-dose (2 mg) or low-dose (1 mg) oral 17β-oestradiol and placebo.

of measurements of oestrogen status, body mass, and serum and urinary markers of bone turnover, they are able to predict fast bone losers[23]. They have followed up three groups of women predicted to be normal, fast or borderline bone losers and by means of serial bone density measurements have been able to confirm the efficacy of their biochemical predictor tests.

Treatment of established osteoporosis (C. Gennari)

Gennari described recent studies carried out by his group on prevention or reversal of bone loss in women with spinal osteoporosis as diagnosed by the presence of spinal fractures or lumbar bone density values more than 2 standard deviations below normal. Each study was placebo controlled and conducted over a period of 12 months. The parameters measured included urinary hydroxyproline, intestinal calcium absorption and lumbar bone density. In the first study, calcium supplementation was without effect, but some slowing of bone loss was seen when lysine was added to improve absorption. Another study showed a beneficial effect on all 3 parameters with conjugated equine oestrogens alone or with ethinyl oestradiol plus a progestogen, while 1,25 dihydroxycholecalciferol had a convincing effect only on calcium absorption. Calcitonin at a high dose had significant beneficial effects on all parameters, while a less frequent dose led to some improvement in bone density. An anabolic steroid, nandrolone decanoate, was also effective in increasing bone density and calcium absorption. Bone biopsy in these cases suggested that this was achieved by increasing bone formation. The results of the studies are summarized in Figure 11.5.

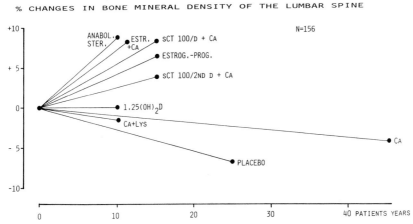

% CHANGES IN BONE MINERAL DENSITY OF THE LUMBAR SPINE

FIGURE 11.5 Cumulative changes in the vertebral bone mineral density of post-menopausal osteoporotics in response to a variety of treatments. (sCT = salmon calcitonin; anabol. ster. = anabolic steroid; Ca = calcium; Lys = lysine)

Conclusion

It is now clear that the menopause is the single most important event in the development of osteoporosis. However, other factors must interact with ovarian hormone deficiency to determine individual susceptibility. With the new techniques of bone mass measurements, particularly dual photon absorptiometry and computed tomography, assessments can be made in the clinically relevant sites in the axial skeleton. Thus, the pronounced and rapid effect of ovarian failure on the skeleton can be clearly demonstrated, and treatment regimens effectively assessed. It is quite clear at present that hormone replacement therapy with oestrogen and progestogen is the most effective proven treatment for the prevention of osteoporosis. The use of calcium is clearly questionable, while the use of calcitonin awaits further evaluation. In the established osteoporotic, positive effects on bone density can be obtained with hormone replacement, calcitonin or anabolic steroid therapy. Conversely, the use of calcium or vitamin D is unable to arrest bone loss.

When considering long-term treatments for the prevention of post-menopausal osteoporosis, it is necessary to bear in mind the potential benefits or risks of the therapies in other areas, such as the cardiovascular system. While oestrogens are beneficial in this respect, care must be taken in the choice of the progestogen. The route of administration for hormone replacement is likely to prove of considerable importance in this respect. With suitable selection of patients and appropriate preventive therapy, it seems likely that a major impact on the reduction of osteoporosis could be achieved in the future.

References

1. Stevenson, J. C., Whitehead, M. I. (1982). Post-menopausal osteoporosis. *Br. Med. J.*, **285**, 585
2. Stevenson, J. C., Banks, I. M., Spinks, T. J. et al. (1987). Regional and total skeletal measurements in the early postmenopause. *J. Clin. Invest.*, **80**, 258
3. Lindsay, R., Aitken, J. M., Anderson, J. B. et al. (1976). Long-term prevention of postmenopausal osteoporosis by oestrogen. *Lancet*, **i**, 1038
4. Richelson, L. S., Wahner, H. W., Melton, L. J. et al. (1984). Relative contributions of aging and estrogen deficiency to postmenopausal bone loss. *N. Engl. J. Med.*, **311**, 1273
5. Garn, S. M. (1970). *The Earlier Gain and Later Loss of Cortical Bone.* (Springfield: C. C. Thomas)
6. Matkovic, V., Kostial, K., Simonovic, I. et al. (1979). Bone status and fracture rates in two regions of Yugoslavia. *Am. J. Clin. Nutr.*, **32**, 540
7. Heany, R. P., Recker, R. R., Saville, P. D. (1978). Menopausal changes in calcium balance performance. *J. Lab. Clin. Med.*, **92**, 953
8. Riggs, B. L., Melton, L. J. (1986). Involutional osteoporosis. *N. Engl. J. Med.*, **314**, 1676
9. Gryfe, C. I., Amies, A., Ashley, M. J. (1977). A longitudinal study of falls in an elderly population: 1. Incidence and morbidity. *Age and Ageing*,

10. Melton, L. J., Riggs, B. L. (1986). Epidemiology and cost of osteoporotic fractures. In *Second International Conference on Osteoporosis. Social and Clinical Aspects*, pp. 23–31. (Milan: Masson Italia Editori)
11. Cameron, J. R., Mazess, R. B., Sorenson, J. A. (1968). Precision and accuracy of bone mineral determination by direct photon absorptiometry. *Invest. Radiol.*, **3**, 141

12. Mazess, R. B., Peppler, W., Chesney, R. W. et al. (1984). Does bone measurement on the radius indicate skeletal status? *J. Nucl. Med.*, **25**, 281

13. Awbrey, B. J., Jacobson, P. C., Grubb, S. A. et al. (1984). Bone density in women: a modified procedure for measurement of distal radial density. *J. Orthop. Res.*, **2**, 321

14. Madsen, M., Peppler, W., Mazess, R. B. (1976). Vertebral and total body bone mineral content by dual photon absorptiometry. In Pors-Neilsen S., Hjorting-Hansen E. (eds.). *Proceedings of 11th European Symposium on Calcified Tissues*, pp. 361–364. (Copenhagen: FADL Publishing)

15. Dunn, W., Wahner, H. W., Riggs, B. L. (1980). Measurement of bone mineral content in human vertebrae and hip by dual photon absorptiometry. *Radiology*, **136**, 485

16. Genant, H. K., Boyd, D. P. (1977). Quantitative bone mineral analysis using dual-energy computed tomography. *Invest. Radiol.*, **12**, 545

17. Laval-Jeantet, A. M., Roger, B., Bouysse, S. et al. (1986). Influence of vertebral fat content on quantitative CT density. *Radiology*, **159**, 463

18. Cann, C. E., Genant, H. K., Kolb, F. O. et al. (1985). Quantitative computed tomography for prediction of vertebral fracture risk. *Metab. Bone Dis. Rel. Res.*, **6**, 1

19. Riggs, B. L., Wahner, H. W., Dunn, W. L. et al. (1981). Differential changes in bone mineral density of the appendicular and axial skeleton with aging. *J. Clin. Invest.*, **67**, 328

20. Christiansen, C., Christensen, M. S., McNair, P. et al. (1980). Prevention of early postmenopausal bone loss: controlled 2-year study in 315 normal females. *Eur. J. Clin. Invest.*, **10**, 273

21. Riis, B., Thomsen, K., Christiansen, C. (1987). Does calcium supplementation prevent postmenopausal bone loss? *N. Engl. J. Med.*, **316**, 173

22. Christiansen C., Christensen, M. S., Transbol, I. (1981). Bone mass in postmenopausal women after withdrawal of oestrogen-gestagen replacement therapy. *Lancet*, **i**, 459

23. Christiansen, C., Riis, B. J., Rodbro, P. (1987). Prediction of rapid bone loss in postmenopausal women. *Lancet*, **i**, 1105

12

Sex hormones and senses

Chairman: P. M. SARREL (USA)
Speakers: P. M. SARREL (USA), L. E. MARKS (USA), S. SCHWARTZ-
GIBLIN (USA)

This workshop comprised three presentations, the first being the introduction by P. Sarrel (Chairman) on the subject of ovarian hormones and the nervous system. The second was a discussion by L. Marks of the theory and techniques of psychophysical measurement, which also included a presentation of preliminary findings relating to vibratory sensitivity and two-point discrimination in menopausal women before and after hormone treatment. In the third, S. Schwartz-Giblin described recent and ongoing experimental work to determine the effects of oestrogen and progesterone on the processing of cutaneous information by the rat spinal cord.

Sarrel summarized the findings of basic research studies showing the effects of ovarian steroids on nerve cell function. Nerve cells at the periphery, in the spinal cord and in the brain have been shown to contain receptors for ovarian steroids[1]. Oestradiol-17β has direct electrical effects on nerve transmission, interacts with nerve cell membranes and enzymes and affects neural deoxyribonucleic acid (DNA) so as to increase or decrease production of ribonucleic acid (RNA) coding for specific proteins[2,3]. Ovarian steroids can increase or decrease the release of neural transmitters. Given such widespread effects by ovarian steroids on nerve cells, it is not surprising to find that the change in ovarian function at the menopause is associated with signs and symptoms of altered nervous system function. Signs of peripheral neuropathy include paresthesia and altered touch perception. Also evident are states of depression and anxiety – including mid-life agoraphobia – which appear to reflect central nervous system changes. Dysfunction of the central thermoregulatory centre is thought to be the cause of 'hot flushes'. Emphasis was laid on the need to be aware of hormone and nerve function studies in animals as a potential guide which might provide insight into human neuropsychiatric problems.

Marks began his presentation by characterizing the role of the senses, i.e. touch, smell, taste, etc. Sensory perception involves a complex set of processes, combining peripheral detection, integration and comparison of the stimulus within the central nervous system, and interpretation. Even the simplest of perceptual tasks can involve several levels of neurological functioning. The application of sensory testing techniques to determine the neurological effects of ovarian steroids must therefore be undertaken in the realization that the findings of any given study may reflect specific changes in either peripheral nerve receptors or central processing neurons, or indeed both.

Detection of a stimulus is the primary task. With this in mind, Marks then went on to emphasize the importance of a forced-choice protocol as a technique to help eliminate confounding factors such as 'response biases' in sensory discrimination. A brief review of the pertinent literature indicated many reports of changes in taste and olfaction as well as in tactile discrimination during the menstrual cycles; such changes may relate to changing levels of ovarian hormones. It appears that vibratory stimulation detected by the corpuscles of Pacini is particularly sensitive to hypo-oestrogenic conditions.

Marks concluded by presenting preliminary findings from a double-blind placebo/oestradiol study currently in progress at Yale. These findings show that vibratory sensitivity to 250 Hertz stimulation (known to be mediated by Pacinian corpuscles) is improved when oestradiol is taken by menopausal women but is unaffected by placebo. Direct correlations were found between changes in vibration threshold and both serum oestradiol levels and follicle-stimulating hormone (FSH) suppression (Figures 12.1 and 12.2). A description was also given of the findings of two-point discrimination tests. To date, two-point sensitivity has not been found to change with hormone replacement therapy, but it should be remembered that these are preliminary results.

Schwartz-Giblin presented the results of new studies on the lordosis response of rats. Lordosis is an essential reproductive behaviour which has been shown to be dependent on both ovarian steroid hormones and cutaneous stimulation of the flanks and perineum.

Firstly a series of experiments were described indicating that progesterone modifies the synaptic activity of a segmental interneuron. Pulses to the pudendal nerve and to the flank skin nerve ordinarily

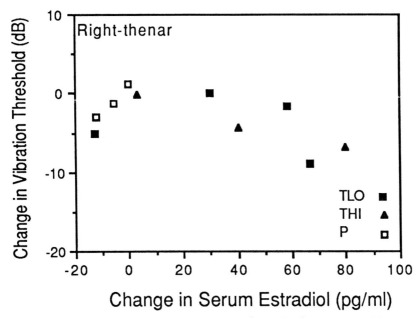

FIGURE 12.1 The difference in vibration thresholds (in decibels) prior to administration of hormone replacement, and 20 weeks after, plotted against the corresponding difference in serum estradiol. The open squares give results for patients receiving placebo patches (P); filled squares and triangles give results, respectively for patients who received low dose oestrogen patches (TLO) and those who received high dose patches (THI). Thresholds were measured in the thenar eminence of each patient's right hand[4,5]. (Placebo/Control Study, Courtesy Dr Lawrence Marks, John Pierce Foundation and Yale University)

lead to action potentials on the motor nerve of the lateral longissimus muscle and then to electromyogram (EMG) activity (Figure 12.3). There is both an early and a late response to stimulation. The late response depends on descending inputs in the anterolateral columns of the spinal cord. These studies revealed that late activity evoked from the flank skin was more probable when animals were primed with oestrogen, thus suggesting that descending inputs may carry hormone information indirectly relayed from the hypothalamus. When the animals were given progesterone a major effect was seen, since the late response was facilitated (Figure 12.4). It was postulated that this might be due to progesterone effects on the neurotransmitter gamma-aminobutyric acid (GABA) and the mechanisms by which it influences spinal cord activity.

In the second part of the presentation, evidence was presented for

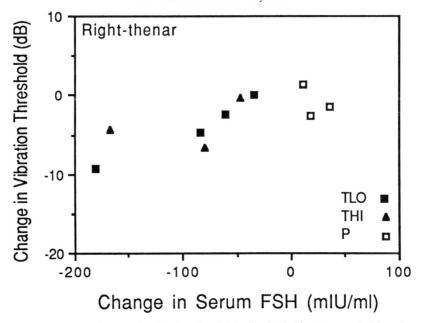

FIGURE 12.2 The difference in vibration thresholds (in decibels) prior to administration of hormone replacement, and 20 weeks after, plotted against the corresponding difference in serum FSH. The open squares give results for patients receiving placebo patches (P); filled squares and triangles give results, respectively for patients who received low dose oestrogen patches (TLO) and those who received high dose patches (THI). Thresholds were measured in the thenar eminence of each patient's right hand[4,5].
(Placebo/Control Study, Courtesy Dr Lawrence Marks, John Pierce Foundation and Yale University)

steroid hormone effects on benzodiazepine (BZD) binding to the GABA/BZD/Chloride receptor in the spinal cord. Oestrogen-concentrating cells are present in the substantia gelatinosa (SG), and in the central canal region of the spinal cord, two areas implicated in sensory integration. Binding studies reveal indications of neurotransmitter activity. Progesterone-enhanced binding occurs in the SG *in vivo*, but not *in vitro*, suggesting that the effect is due to a progesterone metabolite. Pretreatment with oestrogen diminished the progesterone effect. These studies suggest that progesterone is involved in sensory processing, since signals pass through the spinal cord tracts.

The final series of experiments demonstrated a GABA-blockade effect in rats. Intrathecal bicuculline blocked GABA inhibition, leading to a modification in response to light tactile stimulation. A state of hyperalgesia and touch avoidance was induced. Primed with oestrogen

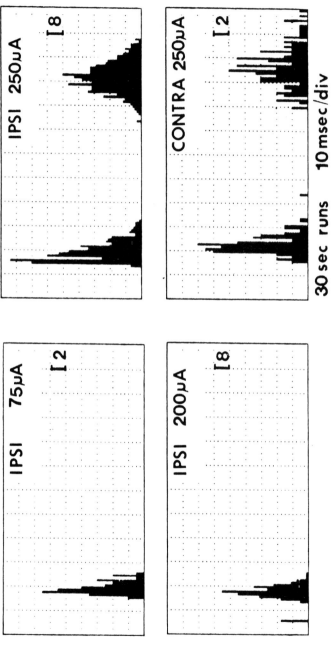

FIGURE 12.3 PST histograms of EMG potentials recorded from lateral longissimus during 30 seconds of stimulation at 2 train/sec to the cutaneous nerve innervating the ipsilateral or contralateral flank. Note the different vertical gain (spikes/div) in each panel. All horizontal divisions are 10 msec. The data is from an oestrogen-primed ovariectomized female rat. (Courtesy Schwartz-Giblin, Rockefeller University)

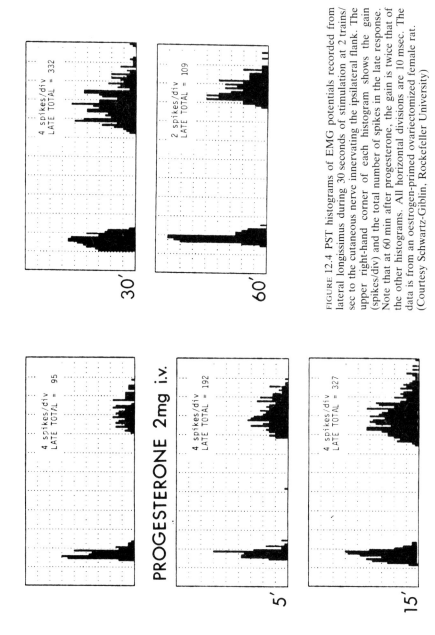

FIGURE 12.4 PST histograms of EMG potentials recorded from lateral longissimus during 30 seconds of stimulation at 2 trains/sec to the cutaneous nerve innervating the ipsilateral flank. The upper right-hand corner of each histogram shows the gain (spikes/div) and the total number of spikes in the late response. Note that at 60 min after progesterone, the gain is twice that of the other histograms. All horizontal divisions are 10 msec. The data is from an oestrogen-primed ovariectomized female rat. (Courtesy Schwartz-Giblin, Rockefeller University)

and progesterone, the rats should have displayed proceptive behaviour patterns. However, the GABA blockade altered the female predisposition to somatosensory stimulation and avoidance behaviour was displayed (Figures 12.5 and 12.6).

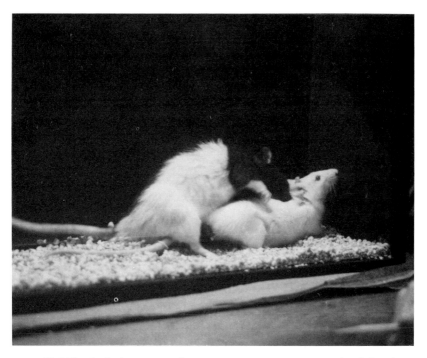

FIGURE 12.5 The lordosis posture of an oestrogen + progesterone primed female rat elicited by the males flank palpation and perineal thrusting during mounting. (Courtesy Schwartz-Giblin, Rockefeller University)

It is clear from work such as this that basic mechanisms in cutaneous sensory processing – in particular those leading to reproductive, lordotic response – involve the spinal cord and are influenced by ovarian steroids. The application of these findings to the understanding of human behaviour remains to be explored. This workshop served to heighten awareness of the importance of neurological changes at the menopause and the potential for hormone replacement to maintain nervous system function.

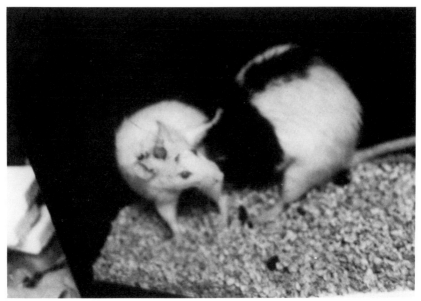

FIGURE 12.6 Avoidance of male reproductive behaviour demonstrated by the albino female rat primed with oestrogen and progesterone within the first 10 minutes following an injection of the GABA antagonist, bicuculline into the lumbar subarachnoid space. (Courtesy Schwartz-Giblin, Rockefeller University)

REFERENCES

1. Pfaff, D. W. (1980). *Estrogens and Brain Function* (New York [USA], Heidelberg, Berlin [West Germany]: Springer-Verlag)
2. Gorski, J., Welshons, W. V., Sakai, D. et al. (1986). Evolution of a model of estrogen action. *Rec. Prog. in Horm. Res.*, **42**, 297
3. McEwen, B. (1986). Ovarian hormone action in the brain: implications for the menopause. In Notelovitz M. and van Keep P. A. (eds.). *The Climacteric in Perspective*, pp. 207–209. (Lancaster: MTP Press)
4. Gescheider, G. A., Verrillo, R. T. (1984). Effects of the menstrual cycle on vibro tactile sensitivity. *Percept. Psychophys.*, **36**, 586
5. Verrillo, R. T. (1980). Age related changes in the sensitivity to vibration. *J. Gerontol.*, **35**, 185

13

Urogenital problems

Chairman: T. RUD (NORWAY)
Speakers: H. REKERS (BELGIUM), A. VICTOR (SWEDEN), E. BORSTAD (NORWAY), A. R. GENAZZANI (ITALY), A. BRANDBERG (SWEDEN), G. HEIMER (SWEDEN)

Rekers presented the results of a postal questionnaire used by his group concerning the prevalence and aetiology of urinary and vaginal symptoms in a random sample of a female population aged between 35 and 80 years in a medium-large Dutch city. This was sent out to 1,900 women and responses were received from 1,299 (68.4%), of whom 27.3% were pre-menopausal, 6.6% peri-menopausal and 66.1% post-menopausal.

As can be seen from Table 13.1 the predominant urogenital·symptom was urinary incontinence (26.3%). Of the women affected, 30.9% had symptoms of urinary stress incontinence only and 7.3% had symptoms of urge incontinence only, while mixed incontinence symptoms were noted in 61.8% of the post-menopausal women.

In 28.1% of the post-menopausal incontinent women the symptoms had started before the climacteric, in 17.5% during the climacteric phase and in 54.4% afterwards.

Table 13.1 (H. REKERS ET AL.)

Urinary symptoms in post-menopausal women	
Incontinence	26.3%
Urgency ($\leq$ 5 min.)	14.9%
Frequency ($\geq$ 7x/day)	19.6%
Nocturia ($\geq$ 2x/night)	17.6%
Dysuria	10.5%
Cystitis during preceding year	10.1%

The prevalence of urinary incontinence by age was found to decrease from age 60 up to age 70, and thereafter to rise with advancing years.

Three independent predisposing factors to incontinence were found:

1. the menopause,
2. previous pelvic surgery, and
3. vaginal childbirth.

It was concluded that significantly more women become incontinent during or shortly after the climacteric than at any other period in life.

Moreover, this relation could not be explained by either possible confounding factors or other predisposing factors.

The Rekers group also found that urinary symptoms are at least as common as vaginal symptoms in post-menopausal women. The vagina and the lower urinary tract tissues share the same embryological origin and many of the lower tissues have been shown to be oestrogen-dependent. Menopause research consequently also needs to focus on symptoms of the urinary tract and the possibilities for treating these with oestrogens.

Before administering treatment to an elderly woman complaining of urogenital problems, the primary investigation should be aimed at correct diagnosis.

Victor pointed out the importance of a gynaecological examination to detect signs of atrophic changes, genital prolapse and tumours. Simple urological tests, neurological tests and measurements of residual urine can be performed concomitantly. In cases of urinary incontinence an accurate case history is of the utmost importance. Questionnaires serve to ensure that no important questions are forgotten, and they may also be of diagnostic value, as might the simple visual analogue scale. He pointed out the importance and necessity of keeping micturition volume and frequency charts to establish an objective assessment of the complaints, such charts being of great diagnostic value.

Standardized short tests have several disadvantages, especially in elderly women. A pad-weighing test performed by the patient at home over 48 hours will not only yield better information on the problems of daily life, but will also help in the choice of protective aids and follow-up treatment.

For an exact diagnosis which meets the criteria of the International

Continence Society, invasive urodynamic investigations are necessary.

In many cases, however, diagnostic accuracy will be sufficiently high to enable treatment to be started without having recourse to such methods.

Borstad drew attention to the results of surgical treatment of urinary stress incontinence (USI) with or without vaginal prolapse in elderly women. She stated that about 25% of patients admitted for prolapse have USI and that about 25% of continent women treated for prolapse suffer from USI after vaginal repair.

A great variety of surgical procedures had been proposed for USI and prolapse, a fact that reflected the difficulty of treating these conditions and might indicate that surgical techniques should be more individualized. In her department all women suffering from prolapse with or without USI, and USI without prolapse, were examined preoperatively and 3 months postoperatively by means of simultaneous urethrocystometry (SUCM) and cysto-urethrography (CURG). This was carried out in the search for parameters to predict the risk of USI after operation in previously continent women and to identify factors during operation that could be responsible for failure to cure or even for causing USI.

USI without prolapse is treated with a modified Burch colposuspension. If the patient also has a genital prolapse, she undergoes vaginal repair with additional Kelly stitches. The overall success rate is about 85% after colposuspension, but it would seem that the younger the patient, the better are the results (Figures 13.1 and 13.2). This might suggest that there are other aetiological factors in the elderly. However, using the same continence parameters (no visible leakage with 300 ml in the bladder during repeated coughing in a standing position), the results after the Manchester procedure showed a cure rate of only 25% and, what was even worse, 25% of the continent women became incontinent after the vaginal repair.

The crucial point in treating and preventing USI after surgery is to reduce the mobility of the bladder neck and the proximal urethra. Preoperative CURG would facilitate the right choice of surgical procedure. Prolapse of the urethra without cystocele should be treated by colposuspension. When it is necessary to carry out a vaginal repair, it is important to ensure proper suspension of the urethra. A cystocele should not be corrected too well and a rectocele should only be

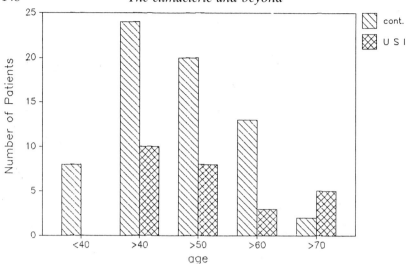

FIGURE 13.1 Results following colposuspension for urinary stress incontinence (USI) – significance of age. (n = 93). (E. Borstad)

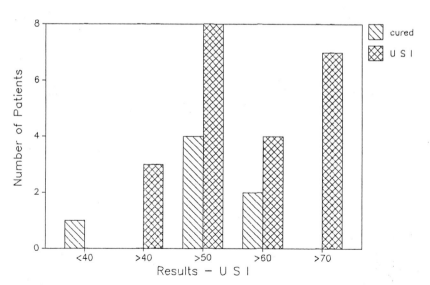

FIGURE 13.2 Results following vaginal repair for urinary incontinence (USI) – significance of age (n = 29). (E. Borstad)

corrected if it is a problem for the patient.

Borstad concluded that surgical treatment of USI should be individualized according to the defect demonstrated by X-ray. Because of the age-dependency of the success rate, she suggested that women aged over 70 should perhaps receive lengthy prior treatment with oestrogens.

Although oestriol has been commercially available as a therapeutic agent for more than four decades, the dosages used and the results obtained have varied considerably in different studies.

Some of the controversy concerning the biological potency of oestriol may be related to the dose and the route of administration.

Genazzani presented the results seen by his group in 29 postmenopausal women suffering from USI and other urinary problems who were treated with vaginal cream containing oestriol (0.5 mg once daily for 4 weeks and then twice weekly for a further 4 weeks). All patients were reassessed after 4 and 8 weeks of treatment (Table 13.2). There was no correlation between clinical outcome and either age or the time interval between menopause and onset of USI. However, the 10 patients who were cured had been suffering from USI for less than one year at the start of the study, whereas the improved and stabilized patients had had their symptoms for a considerably longer period.

Although most clinicians have the impression that oestriol has a beneficial effect in treating elderly women with urogenital problems, it

Table 13.2 (A. R. GENAZZANI ET AL.) RESULTS IN 29 POST-MENOPAUSAL WOMEN TREATED WITH VAGINAL CREAM CONTAINING OESTRIOL (0.5 MG DAILY FOR 4 WEEKS, THEN TWICE WEEKLY FOR 4 WEEKS)

	Affected patients	Cured No	%	Improved No	%	Stabilized No	%
USI	19	10	53	5	26	4	21
Atrophy	9	4	44	5	56	–	–
Sensory urgency	8	3	37	3	37	2	25
Nycturia	6	2	33	3	50	1	17
Frequency > 10 times/day	6	5	83	1	17	–	–

is the workshop chairman's opinion that controlled studies to evaluate oestriol versus placebo are still lacking in the scientific literature.

An effort to remedy this situation was made by *Heimer*, who treated 40 post-menopausal patients in a geriatric hospital suffering from urogenital disorders with oestriol for 6 weeks. These women had symptoms of vaginal atrophy, urge and mixed incontinence, as well as recurrent tract infections. None of the patients had received oestrogen treatment previously.

To exclude women with a proliferative endometrium, 5 mg medroxyprogesterone acetate was given once a day for 7 days starting two weeks prior to the oestrogen treatment. Since no vaginal bleeding occurred in any of the women, all were allowed to continue in the study. The progestogen test was repeated after termination of the oestriol treatment.

A dose of 0.5 mg oestriol was administered intravaginally every day for the first two weeks. Thereafter, the women were randomly allocated to either 0.5 mg oestriol once or twice weekly for a further four weeks. Gynaecological examinations were performed four times during the trial: before the oestrogen therapy was started, then after 1, 2 and finally 6 weeks of treatment. The oestrogen influence on the vaginal and urethral epithelium was assessed by means of the Karyopyknotic Index (KPI). In addition, the degree of maturation of the vaginal epithelium was estimated visually and urinary bacteria were cultivated.

A pronounced and progressive rise in KPI was seen in both the vaginal and urethral epithelium during daily treatment with oestriol. However, neither of the two subsequent maintenance doses were sufficient to maintain the initial maturation of the vaginal and urethral epithelium induced by oestriol, since the KPI values fell back to pretreatment levels within the further 4-week treatment period. The visual assessment overestimated the oestriol effect induced in the vaginal epithelium, while no changes in urinary bacteria were observed. None of the women experienced withdrawal bleeding after the progestogen challenge test following the oestriol treatment.

Heimer concluded that the trial yielded no evidence to indicate that elderly patients in geriatric hospitals need lower doses of oestriol than those commonly used for the treatment of urogenital disorders in post-menopausal women. A higher maintenance dose than that administered in this study would seem to be needed to maintain the maturation of the vaginal and urethral epithelium.

Brandberg, as a bacteriologist, had studied the use of antibiotics and changes in the vaginal flora in 41 elderly women (aged between 80 and 90 years) in a geriatric hospital before and after treatment with oestriol tablets. In pre-menopausal women, the presence of oestrogens maintains a normotrophic vaginal epithelium which produces the glucogen required by the Döderlein lactobacilli. The lactic acid keeps the pH at about 4, thus maintaining a physiological vaginal flora. In post-menopausal women in whom no glycogen is produced owing to the lack of oestrogens, the Döderlein lactobacilli will disappear, resulting in a more alcaline pH (range 5–6) which will facilitate the invasion of gram-negative bacteria. Thus, elderly women are more prone to bacterial colpitis and cystitis.

Brandberg followed up 41 patients for 6 months before and after oestriol treatment. Initially, a 'starter' dose of 3 mg/day oestriol was administered orally for 30 days, after which a maintenance dose of 1 mg/day was given. The faecal bacterial type was dominant in the vagina before treatment with oestriol, whereas lactobacilli predominated after the oestriol treatment. A gynaecological examination revealed that after oestriol treatment the vaginal mucosa became thickened and well-vascularized, with good secretion. Some urogenital disorders are in fact more probably caused by an atrophic mucosa than by true infection.

Urogenital infections expressed in terms of the number of weeks on antibiotic treatment were reduced to 0.7% as compared with 11% in the non-oestriol-treated patients.

Although oestrogen treatment would seem to play a very important role in reducing urogenital problems in the elderly, it should always be remembered that patients in institutions or hospitals are more prone to get infection than women in the general population.

Consequently, apart from the need to give oestrogens to prevent urinary tract infections and symptoms caused by mucosal atrophy of the vagina, it is also important to keep patients active and to make minimum use of indwelling catheters (pads should be used instead of catheters in incontinent patients).

In summary, urogenital problems are very common in elderly women. Many of the complaints suffered might be due to oestrogen deficiency, but not all disorders respond to oestrogen treatment. From this point of view oestrogen therapy has no place during the fertile years while there is sufficient oestrogen production. Urogenital problems and climacteric symptoms (hot flushes, etc.) are best treated with oestradiol and isolated urogenital problems with a less systemically potent oestrogen, i.e. oestriol.

Should oestriol be administered vaginally or orally? It should be remembered that, when given orally, oestriol is a short-acting oestrogen which is rapidly conjugated in the liver. About one-third to one-half of the circulating oestrogens are secreted into the bile, and from this fraction 80% is reabsorbed after hydrolysis by bacterial beta-glycoronidase in the intestinal tract.

In addition to enterohepatic recirculation, the intestinal microflora as well as the mucosal cell metabolism must also therefore be considered as important for the metabolism and reabsorption of oestriol from the intestine.

It is the workshop chairman's opinion that oestriol, if given orally, 3 mg/day for the first 2–3 weeks, should be followed by a maintenance dose of 1–2 mg/day. According to Heimer, such administration of oestriol in the morning resulted in an early plasma oestriol rise within 3–4 hours. The mean plasma oestriol level then remained stable for another 4 hours after which it decreased slowly to almost the pretreatment value after 24 hours.

However, when oestriol was given vaginally, either in the morning or at bedtime, ,there was no difference in its 24-hour systemic availability (area under the curve). Hence, the therapeutic effect of intravaginal oestriol can be expected to be equally good whether it is administered in the morning or in the evening. A minimal plasma oestriol elevation seems to be induced by the intake of food after both morning and evening vaginal administration of oestriol, possibly due to enterohepatic recirculation.

The workshop chairman is of the opinion that when oestriol is administered vaginally, 0.5 mg should be given daily for 2–3 weeks, followed by a maintenance dose of 0.5 mg every second day.

As in the case of other hormone-deficit symptoms, oestriol should most probably also be given lifelong.

As regards side effects, elderly women with atrophic vaginal mucosa might experience soreness and 'worsening' of their symptoms during the first few weeks of vaginally administered oestriol. However, when the mucosal membrane becomes more trophic these symptoms usually disappear. As for more serious side effects, there is no evidence to indicate that oestriol at the abovementioned dose will give rise to thromboembolic complications or oestrogen-dependent cancers.

Conclusion

Urogenital problems are very common in the elderly woman. Urinary urgency, slight or moderate urinary stress incontinence, dysuria and recurrent urinary cystitis can be expected to be reduced after oestriol treatment. This treatment can be administered vaginally or orally. However, before starting any treatment at all, it is essential to obtain a detailed history and carry out a physical examination.

14

Psychosocial models of the climacteric

Chairman: J. G. GREENE (UK)
Co-chair: M. LOCK (CANADA)
Speakers: S. BALLINGER (AUSTRALIA), M. HUNTER (UK), J. RESNICK
(USA), A. HOLTE (NORWAY), M. LOCK (CANADA)

Introduction

Until relatively recently much of the psychosocial research on the
climacteric was descriptive or empirical in nature. This was only to be
expected in such a relatively new scientific discipline, since early researchers were concerned mainly with establishing certain basic facts
(e.g. the prevalence of different psychological symptoms at the menopause) and with laying down a data base.

During the past 5–6 years, however, two noticeable trends have
become apparent. Firstly, researchers are increasingly examining
aetiological relationships between variables from different *domains*
and, secondly, in doing so they are making increasing use of *methods*
and *concepts* derived from other areas of psychosocial research[1,2].

This means that psychosocial research on the climacteric is becoming
more theory oriented than hitherto and research design more complex
and sophisticated. At this stage in the development of a science,
researchers begin to construct conceptual models, either explicitly or
implicitly. If their approach is explicit, this usually entails producing a
diagrammatic representation of the proposed causal relationships between a set of constructs, the constructs being derived from operation-
al measures and the relationships from empirically established associations between these measures. This, however, is an exercise which is
heavily influenced by the researcher's own perspective on and
approach to the subject matter.

It therefore seemed opportune at this point in time to bring together a group of researchers currently engaged in this form of research activity and to ask them to think explicitly about their own research in such terms. In this way it was hoped to compare and contrast, and perhaps even establish links between the different models that are currently emerging.

The models

Ballinger opened the proceedings by outlining what could be called a 'stress-vulnerability' model. The assumption on which her research is based is that hormonal changes at the menopause can cause not only physical and emotional symptoms, but also make women more vulnerable to the effects of stress. Thus, stress and the menopause, both of which can produce the same or similar symptoms, can also interact to exacerbate these symptoms. Ballinger illustrated her approach with examples of findings from two research studies. The general methodology of this research can be found elsewhere[3].

In the first study the relationships between various hormonal measures (e.g. urinary cortisol, plasma oestradiol, etc.) and stress scores (life events, stress/coping ratings) were compared in a patient and a non-patient group.

Higher and more significant correlations between high stress scores, anxiety and depression ratings and lowered biochemical measures were found in the patient group than in the non-patient group. These patterns of correlations are shown in Table 14.1. Furthermore, when groups were combined and subjects classified according to whether they scored high or low on each of the clinical ratings, significant intergroup differences were found in oestrogen and cortisol levels. A consistent association was thus established between psychosocial and hormonal variables.

In the second study Ballinger followed up a group of 400 women who attended a multidisciplinary menopause clinic and compared the women's own reports on the problems presented and treatment received with those of the clinic staff. A number of discrepancies emerged between patient and staff perceptions of what had transpired.

Notable among these differences were contradictions in the perception of hypothalamic and psychological symptoms between patients, psychologists and gynaecologists. There were also discrepancies in the memories of women as regards the professional help they had received

Table 14.1 PEARSON PRODUCT MOMENT CORRELATION COEFFICIENTS BETWEEN LOGGED BIOCHEMICAL MEASURES AND CLINICAL STRESS SCORES IN THE PATIENT AND NON-PATIENT GROUPS

	Patient group				*Non-patient group*			
	N	*Stress rating*	*Depression rating*	*Anxiety rating*	*N*	*Stress rating*	*Depression rating*	*Anxiety rating*
Cortisol	70	0.10	0.05	0.09	120	0.05	0.14	0.14
Urinary E_1	66	0.13	0.40****	0.40****	120	0.18**	0.12	0.14
Urinary E_2	66	0.11	0.39****	0.39****	120	0.08	0.09	0.08
Urinary E_3	66	0.10	0.33****	0.36****	120	0.30****	0.21***	0.23**
Urinary $E_1+E_2+E_3$	66	0.12	0.40****	0.41****	120	0.21****	0.16**	0.17*
Urinary 20HE1	72	0.19*	0.31****	0.33****	116	0.14	0.03	0.01
Urinary 20HE	72	0.19*	0.22*	0.19*	116	0.09	0.033	0.020
Plasma E_1	95	0.07	0.06	0.06	141	0.10	0.06	0.08
Plasma E_1S	94	0.03	0.02	0.02	141	0.01	0.01	0.09
Plasma E_2	95	0.35****	0.33****	0.32****	135	0.01	0.05	0.05
Total plasma $E_1+E_1S+E_2$	92	0.19*	0.15	0.15	135	0.10	0.03	0.12

$* = P < 0.05$, $** = P < 0.02$, $*** = P < 0.005$, $**** = P < 0.001$

Note: All significant correlations are in the negative direction.

and as regards the psychologist's rating of the stress they were experiencing. Thus there were clear differences in the patients' perceptions of the types of problems they bring to menopause clinics and those of the health professionals who treat them.

Figure 14.1 shows Ballinger's final model of the relationship between psychosocial stress, symptoms and oestrogen levels in the form of a flow diagram. This is presented as a 'reverberating circuit' which can be responsible for the maintenance of symptoms over time. The crucial role of cognitions in this scheme should be noted.

This, of course, raises the general question of the part played by the way in which women perceive symptoms and other events surrounding the menopause, an issue which forms the central theme of the second speaker's research. *Hunter's* starting point is that it is cognition

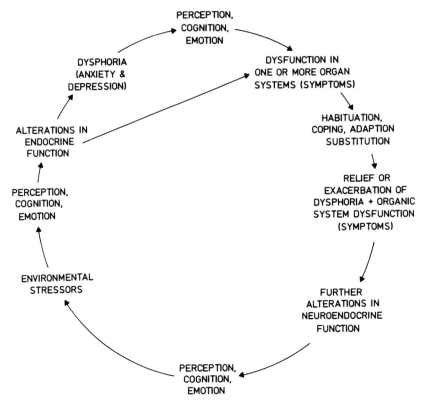

FIGURE 14.1 Model of the role of psychosocial stress in climacteric symptoms and lowered oestrogen levels. (Ballinger)

(thoughts, attitudes, beliefs, explanations) which affect interpretation of events and influence reactions to them. She argues that the incorporation of cognitive factors into models might clarify our understanding of the connection between predictive factors, e.g. life events, and actual experience of the menopause. Hunter gave two illustrative examples of this from her own work, the general methodology of which can be found elsewhere[4].

In a postal survey of 850 women aged 45–65 years with a 3-year follow up of 56 women, a number of questions on stereotypes and beliefs about the menopause were included in the research protocol.

As in other studies, stereotype proved to be more negative than later reported experience of the menopause. However, as can be seen from Table 14.2, negative stereotype nevertheless predicted depressed mood in the peri-menopause and post-menopause. The multiple regression analysis carried out to examine the predictive value of stereotype relative to other factors shows that pre-menopausal depression was the best predictor of depression during menopause. In addition, negative stereotype was not associated with current mood state. On the basis of a cognitive interpretation of these data, some women may hold negative beliefs about the menopause which are relatively independent of depression. This may lead to negative interpretations of physical change and inappropriate attribution of depressed mood to the menopause. Other women, however, who are depressed both before and after the menopause may also interpret changes with a negative bias

Table 14.2 PREDICTING DEPRESSED MOOD: A PROSPECTIVE STUDY

N = 47 (86% response rate)			
(i) *Simple regression analysis*			
Pre-menopause		*Peri/post-menopause*	
Stereotype → r = 0.36 p < 0.02 → Depression			
(ii) *Stepwise multiple regression analysis*			
Predictive factor (pre)	*Beta*	*Correlation*	*%Variance*
Depressed mood	0.42	0.58	34
Stereotype (negative)	0.21	0.36	6
Employment	−0.27	−0.32	5
Socioeconomic status	−0.24	−0.18	6

because of the way the depressed state affects the thinking processes.

In her second example, Hunter reported that women who sought medical help were characterized by two specific beliefs, namely that the menopause is uncontrollable and that it is psychologically upsetting. The holding of these beliefs was also a characteristic that distinguished a clinic sample from a non-clinic sample. The main characteristics of such women were that they tended to report having suffered from premenstrual tension and that they generally had a negative view of their own health. The cognitive interpretation of this is that there is an interplay between experience of premenstrual tension and the development of certain attitudes about aspects of the menstrual cycle, i.e. that it is uncontrollable and is associated with both psychological and physical change. There is also good evidence that it is more difficult to cope with events that are perceived as uncontrollable.

Figure 14.2 depicts this model in general terms. In the light of modern cognitive therapy this model has some direct practical implications. Firstly, in attempts to counter negative stereotypes, Hunter considers that it may be productive to identify and deal with specific beliefs, e.g. regarding controllability and psychological experiences. Secondly, helping women cope with menstrual problems before the menopause might in turn help them feel more positive about coping during the menopause itself.

The third speaker, *Resnick*, broadened the issue in adopting a life-span or life-development approach to the climacteric years. However, as she pointed out, study of the life course presents some problems for the human sciences as now constituted, since each discipline has claimed as its own special domain one aspect only of life, such as personality, social role, or biological functioning, and has generally neglected others [5]. What is required is an interdisciplinary perspective in order to develop a comprehensive model of the climacteric which acknowledges both the psychosocial and the biological markers that characterize adult development during these years. The question raised by Resnick concerns the nature of the processes (biological, psychological and social) that produce psychological change and the way in which they interact.

In her research strategy Resnick sets about answering this question by utilizing factor analysis. This mathematical technique allows a large number of diverse variables to be reduced to a limited number of

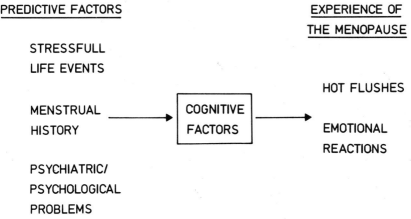

EXPERIENCE OF
THE MENOPAUSE

STRESSFULL
LIFE EVENTS

HOT FLUSHES

MENSTRUAL
HISTORY

COGNITIVE
FACTORS

EMOTIONAL
REACTIONS

PSYCHIATRIC/
PSYCHOLOGICAL
PROBLEMS

FIGURE 14.2 Model of cognitive factors as mediators. (Hunter)

factors or groupings. A total of 27 such variables covering several domains, such as health, psychosocial adaptation and hormonal status, were measured in a group of 137 women aged 36–75 and submitted to a factor analysis using varimax rotation. In all, 8 factors were identified with eigenvalues greater than 1.0. The first and largest of these factors, which had 12 contributory variables, was labelled 'Functional age/ Climacteric'.

This factor is shown in Table 14.3. As can be seen it includes variables from all domains, although the main contributions come from hormonal status and physical health variables. Table 14.4, on the other hand, shows a factor which covers only a single domain, namely psychosocial adaptation. Other factors to emerge were size and fitness, a psychosomatic factor, hospitalization, two hormonally-related factors and a sexual-activity factor.

Resnick argues that the fact that so many of the eight factors which emerged in her study spanned at least two domains confirms the value of continuing with an interdisciplinary approach to future research in this area. She is also of the view that as the knowledge base regarding the climacteric years continues to evolve and explanatory models are postulated, sophisticated design and analysis techniques will need to be developed to handle the overall complexity.

This last point is well illustrated by the work of the fourth speaker, *Holte*, whose research is indeed both sophisticated and complex. Holte

Table 14.3

Factor 1 –	Functional age/Climacteric
Follicle-stimulating hormone	0.90
Menstrual status	0.90
Oestradiol	−0.86
Luteinizing hormone	0.82
Chronological age	0.74
Oestrone	−0.69
Cholesterol	0.60
Androstenedione	−0.57
Dihydrotestosterone	−0.48
Testosterone	−0.45
Arterial blood pressure	0.38
Perceptual speed	−0.34

Table 14.4

Factor 2 –	Psychosocial adaptation
Self concept	0.76
Life satisfaction	0.72
Depression	0.70
Psychosocial adjustment	0.69

reported on the most recent findings that have emerged from the Norwegian Climacteric Project, the major part of which is a longitudinal study being carried out in a large population of 2,400 women in Oslo. Initial cross-sectional analysis confirmed many of the findings of the earlier study carried out in Drammen[6], such as the fact that earlier menstrual coping style predicts many later menopausal complaints, that negative expectations contribute to all types of symptoms, that contrary to the findings in other countries, socioeconomic status has little association with menopausal complaints in Norway, and that the amount of cigarette smoking increases the probability of vasomotor symptoms, this last being a particularly striking observation.

In the prospective part of this study, a randomly selected subsample of 200 pre-menopausal women aged 45–55 at inception were followed up over a four-year period from 1982–86. Each year data were collected on symptoms, psychological testing, social situation, life events and gynaecological examinations. The data obtained are being analyzed by a sophisticated Path Analysis method which examines the strength and direction of the relationship between different variables over time. Figure 14.3 is an example of just one of these types of analysis over the years 1982, 1983 and 1984, showing the strength of the relationship between three variables both in and across these years. Life events include deaths and illnesses of family members, unemployment, and financial and marital problems.

On the basis of these findings Holte has constructed the model shown in Figure 14.4, in which the various pre-existing psychosocial factors, mediated by negative expectations, are depicted as interacting with the menopause, pre-menopausal symptoms and current life events to produce the full-blown climacteric-symptom picture.

A sociocultural perspective

The final speaker, *Lock*, provided a commentary on model building from an anthropological perspective. One of the functions of anthropological research is to take theories and models constructed in the West and test them out cross-culturally. However, as Lock pointed out, while the foregoing models all provide stimulating insights into the complexities of a quantitative approach in which account is taken of

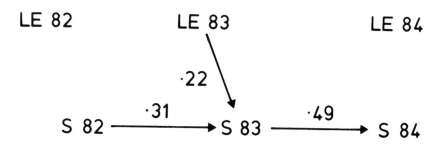

FIGURE 14.3 Path diagram for depression. Symptoms (S) by earlier symptoms (S), life events (LE) and menopausal status (M). (Holte)

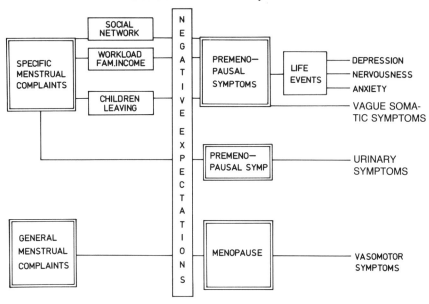

FIGURE 14.4 An integrative model of menopausal complaints. (Holte)

both biological and psychosocial variables, the picture becomes even more complex when the possible application of these models in cross-cultural research is considered.

A number of immediate problems arise. One is that universality of biological functioning cannot be assumed, since there may be considerable variation in, for example, oestrogen levels both between and within populations. Apart from possible variation due to genetics and diet, there is probably considerable variation due to reproductive history. The second major difficulty arises from what is considered 'normal' at the social and psychological levels. Local expectations, meanings and stereotypes associated with the menopause will have a marked effect on the actual experience. These factors need to be taken into account particularly when designing and using measuring instruments. The manner in which people report somatic sensation and symptoms, for example, is profoundly influenced by early socialization, language and social contexts. A third problem concerns the subtle relationship between biological and social functioning. Biology is not a determined basal structure with a veneer of culture spread over it. It has a dynamic and dialectical relationship with culture in which biology is modified by culture and culture constrained by biology.

Lock then went on to consider some ways of at least partially resolving some of the difficulties of cross-cultural model building. One, arising from Hunter's paper, is to build cognitive ratings into instruments or scales. In addition, in applying scales and questionnaires a first step is to collect ethnographic data and subjective accounts of the menopause and then modify instruments in the light of the information obtained. Study also needs to focus on the subjective, descriptive level, not only of symptoms, but also of the social and cultural meaning of the event. For elaboration of these and other cross-cultural issues see Kaufert[7]. Nevertheless, the pervasive influence of cultural factors is such that Lock concluded by casting some doubt on whether a universal model of the climacteric experience is attainable, arguing that perhaps different types of models are required for different purposes.

Discussion

The aim of this Workshop was to compare and contrast, and perhaps establish links between the different psychosocial models of the climacteric that have emerged in recent years. In the course of the discussion between the panel and the audience, following the formal presentations, it became clear that despite the diversity of the approaches and material presented, there was considerably more agreement between speakers than there were differences. Indeed, it was a relatively simple task to establish links between models, and those differences that did exist were more a matter of emphasis than of substance. Some examples of this consensus are given below.

Resnick's interdisciplinary perspective pointed up the need for a multifactorial approach. This was echoed in the work of all the speakers, each of whom incorporate variables from different domains into their research design, and in particular attempt with some success to begin bridging the gap between the biomedical and the psychosocial. Ballinger's emphasis on stress also finds its counterpart in the work of all the others, and it is clear that stressful life events, whether they be long-standing or of recent onset, must be seen as a major contributory factor to women's experience of the menopause.

Again, Hunter's use of cognitions as a mediating variable between psychosocial predictors, such as life events, and experience of the menopause is widespread in the work of others and is given a central role in their final models. Holte's particular contribution is to draw attention to the role of previous patterns of behaviour in shaping the menopausal experience, such as earlier menstrual coping style, and to demonstrate the subtle interaction of variables over time in his prospective study. There is no need to look far to find these themes in the models of others. Also implicit in each model is the notion of vulnerability, since all research indicates that as only some or a minority of women experience serious difficulties during the climacteric, the general thrust of research must be to identify the psychosocial factors that render women vulnerable at that time of life.

As has been observed above, differences between models are largely ones of emphasis. Nevertheless, there are differences in some respects which reflect the sociocultural differences that exist between even the Western populations considered by the speakers. An obvious example here is Holte's finding that social class has little influence on symptoms, which is contrary to that of previous studies and reflects the social homogeneity of Scandinavian society. Differences of this sort clearly point up Lock's admonitions regarding the cultural relativity of models.

Clinical implications

As was noted in the introduction, a model is a simplified representation of the proposed causal relationship between a set of constructs. Such a definition might suggest that models are no more than abstruse theoretical generalizations. This is far from the truth. Models have two important practical functions, in addition to that of specifying the nature and direction of causal relationships. The first is that they provide guidelines for future research, as was amply demonstrated in this Workshop, the second being that they provide guidelines for clinical practice. In the light of the foregoing models these are, to mention but a few: that the help and advice required by a climacteric woman must be provided within the framework of a multidisciplinary team approach; that the nature of all the woman's presenting symptoms and complaints must be clearly specified; that it is necessary to go beyond symptoms and identify the problems, whether recent or longstanding, that may be giving rise to the symptoms; that the woman's personal perception of and the meaning she attaches to events and experiences must be given due consideration; that an adequate history must include information on how she has coped or failed to cope with previous adversity, particularly during other critical phases of her life; and, finally, that all this must be evaluated in the context of her total sociocultural milieu.

Each of the above guidelines highlights a feature of one or other of the models described in this Workshop. It is perhaps the responsibility of the clinician to construct the truly integrative model in the person of the individual woman.

REFERENCES

1. Greene, J. G. (1984). *The Social and Psychological Origins of the Climacteric Syndrome.* (Aldershot, UK; Brookfield, USA: Gower Publishing Company)
2. Severne, L. and Greene, J. G. (1986). Lifestyles; coping with life events and stress at the climacteric. In Notelovitz M. and van Keep P. A. (eds.). *The Climacteric in Perspective.* (Lancaster: MTP Press)
3. Ballinger, S. (1985). Psychosocial stress and symptoms of menopause: a comparative study of menopause clinic patients and non-patients. *Maturitas,* **7**, 315
4. Hunter, M., Battersby, R. and Whitehead, M. (1986). Relationships between psychological symptoms, somatic complaints and menopausal status. *Maturitas,* **8**, 217
5. Levison, D. J. (1986). A conception of adult development. *Am. Psychol.,* **41**, 3
6. Holte, A. and Mikkelsen, A. (1982). Menstrual coping style, social background and climacteric symptoms. *Psychiatry and Soc. Sci.,* **2**, 41
7. Kaufert, P. (1986). Menopause research: The Korpilampi Workshop. *Soc. Sci. and Med.,* **22**, 1285

15

Alternative delivery systems for steroid hormones

Chairwoman: R. SITRUK-WARE (FRANCE)
Speakers: R. SITRUK-WARE (FRANCE), L. FÅHRAEUS (SWEDEN), W. H. UTIAN (USA), A. VICTOR (SWEDEN), J. W. W. STUDD (UK)

Introduction

In 1987 the world population reached the five billion mark and it is expected to rise to six billion by as early as the beginning of the next century.

In parallel to this dramatic population growth, life expectancy is also increasing very fast in both the developed and the developing world. By the year 2025, some 23% of the population in the developed countries and 12% in the developing ones will be aged 60 or over[1].

Among the many great difficulties to which these changes will give rise, the menopause will become a major problem that will no longer be restricted to Western societies.

Of the major menopause-related health disorders, osteoporosis and bone fracture risk will assume an overwhelming importance in both developed and developing communities.

The potential benefits of oestrogen replacement therapy (ERT) for menopausal women are well recognized[2,3] and their preventive effect in regard to osteoporosis has been clearly demonstrated[4]. Improved knowledge of side effects and their mechanisms has led to substantial improvements in therapeutic regimens.

Among the drawbacks ascribed to ERT, endometrial hyperplasia and carcinoma risks still constitute the basis of the arguments advanced by its opponents. However, there is a considerable body of biochemical, experimental and epidemiological evidence to show that these risks are related to an absence of progestational balance[5,6].

Indeed, most scientists involved in menopause research now agree that sequential progestogen addition to ERT will solve the problem of cellular risk.

The relation of cardiovascular risk to ERT still leads to conflicting results[7,8]. Epidemiological studies probably yield opposing data because case-control studies reflect only the effects of past use of oral synthetic oestrogens.

Up to now no prospective epidemiological studies have been initiated to compare the risk in menopausal women treated by traditional ERT methods with that in women treated with new systems of delivering natural oestrogens by other than oral routes.

Metabolic disturbances have in fact been related to synthetic oral oestrogens as well as to increased vascular risk[9]. Both the so-called natural conjugated oestrogens and the synthetic oestrogens have been shown to increase plasma triglycerides (TG) and very-low-density lipoprotein (VLDL)[10,11], to impair several coagulation factors[12], to decrease antithrombin III (AT III) activity[13], to increase plasma renin substrate (RS)[13,14] and presumably to enhance vascular morbidity in non-selected populations[15].

Also, oestrone (E_1) binds preferentially to the liver receptor sites[16] and appears to be twice as active as oestradiol (E_2) as regards liver side effects[17]. Unfortunately, when administered orally, all the other available natural oestrogens are rapidly metabolized in the liver, leading to high circulating levels of E_1 and to an inversion of the E_2/E_1 ratio[18]. Oral administration of micronized E_2 does not solve the problem, giving rise to tremendously increased plasma levels of E_1[19,20] and the same effect is observed after oral ingestion of oestradiol valerate[18,19]. Thus, following oral therapy, the bolus of oestrogens reaching the portal vein and the conversion of E_2 into E_1 in the gut transform the liver cell into a preferential target.

It has consequently been suggested that these hepatocellular effects may be related not only to the type of oestrogen used, but also to the route of administration. Oral therapy actually results in a large, unphysiological bolus of oestrogens being delivered into the portal circulation, whereas in a physiological state oestrogens are secreted into the circulation and delivered to the target organs before they reach the liver.

Alternative delivery systems for steroid administration have accordingly been sought to avoid the so-called first-pass liver effect and so avoid excessive stimulation of liver enzymes and metabolism.

The main goal of pharmaceutical research has been to achieve therapeutic improvement by discovering new galenic formulations able to provide sustained, efficient plasma levels of steroids and in particular of oestradiol.

If we consider conventional galenic preparations (whether administered orally or intravenously) the curve of the plasma levels will first show a peak concentration and then a decrease towards initial pretreatment levels. Plasma concentrations therefore range from the potentially toxic to the ineffective, with considerable inter-individual and intra-individual variations (Figure 15.1)[21].

Repeated administration throughout the day could maintain high, efficient plasma values but this is impractical and nocturnal intakes are not possible.

However, controlled sustained release from long-acting delivery systems would solve the problems of both constancy of plasma levels and acceptability.

What then are the alternatives to oral therapy?

The different controlled-release systems available to deliver oestrogens include transdermal or percutaneous systems, transmucosal delivery via vaginal rings or vaginal creams, and implants.

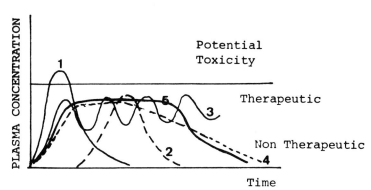

1. CONVENTIONAL
2. DELAYED
3. REPEATED ADMINISTRATION
4. LONG ACTING
5. SUSTAINED RELEASE

FIGURE 15.1 Plasma concentrations obtained with different controlled-release systems (adapted from Segot-Chicq, S. et al.[21])

All of these systems are able to ensure a sustained therapeutic effect for intervals of from 24 hours to several days and to maintain adequate plasma levels over lengthy periods to provide therapeutic efficacy while avoiding peak effects and metabolic drawbacks.

Oral therapy

The oral oestrogens most commonly used are conjugated equine oestrogens and a micronized form of 17 β-oestradiol. The latter provides pre-menopausal levels of oestradiol but gives rise to unphysiological levels of oestrone. A proportion of the administered steroid is initially metabolized within the gut wall and oestradiol is preferentially converted to oestrone[22].

The steroid is then transported to the liver via the portal circulation and further metabolism results in the formation of oestrone sulphate and oestrone glucuronide[23].

One-third of the total administered dose of oestradiol is metabolized in these ways before the systemic circulation is reached[9] and only small increases in plasma levels of E_2 are obtained. Oestradiol has to be given in large doses in order to achieve therapeutic plasma concentrations, but this results in high E_1 plasma levels and supraphysiological amounts of total circulating oestrogens ($E_2 + E_1$ + oestrone glucuronide). It has been estimated that after oral oestrogen therapy the plasma levels of oestrone sulphate are sufficiently high to sustain back conversion to oestrone for many days, thereby potentially maintaining a stimulus for continued endometrial proliferation[24].

Moreover, the high levels of oestrogens reaching the portal vein transform the liver into a preferential target. Oestrone binds preferentially to the liver receptor sites[16] and appears to be twice as active as E_2 as regards liver side effects[17]. Hence, it has been demonstrated that hepatocellular modifications occur after oral therapy whatever the type of oestrogen used, whether conjugated oestrogens or natural 17β-oestradiol[10,13,25].

Another explanation for the enhanced hepatic action of oral oestrogens lies in the preferential uptake of some oestrogens by the liver as compared with other tissues. It has recently been shown that the uptake of some circulating unconjugated and conjugated oestrogens by the liver is much greater than that by the uterus during their passage through the microvascular beds of these two organs[26].

It has also been demonstrated by *in vivo* techniques that the hepatic microvasculature is freely permeable to all oestrogens. Even in the presence of plasma proteins, the extraction of all oral oestrogens in the liver significantly exceeded that in the brain and uterus[27]. These findings provide a further explanation for the enhanced response of hepatic markers of oestrogen action to the oral preparations used in ERT.

Consequently, alternatives to the oral route of administration have been sought in order to bypass the liver.

Percutaneous absorption of oestradiol

The ability of the skin to absorb steroids has been recognized since the beginning of this century and has been extensively studied[28,29]. The use of appropriate vehicles allows penetration through the stratum corneum, which performs the principal 'barrier' function of the epidermis[28]. Different processes occur in sequence. Firstly, the molecules are absorbed within the stratum corneum, secondly, they are retained in the stratum corneum (reservoir effect) and, thirdly, they diffuse through the epidermis and papillary dermis until they reach the capillary plexus and are transferred to the circulating blood. Each step in this chain of events is essential and individual variations at any stage can influence the rate of absorption[28].

Steroids penetrate the stratum corneum quite easily from an appropriated polar vehicle allowing permeation[28]. The steroid-reservoir function of human skin is localized in the stratum corneum, as was demonstrated by Vickers[30]. This reservoir action by the stratum corneum provides a sustained release of percutaneously applied steroid which extends over more than 24 hours.

When applied to human skin in an alcohol solution, oestradiol rapidly penetrates the stratum corneum (within 10 minutes of application). Then diffusion of the steroid through the epidermis and dermis occurs via the pathway described above over a period of several hours[28,31]. The rate of absorption depends upon the dose that is topically applied; about 10% of the total dose passes through the cutaneous barrier, is transferred to the vascular system, and is eliminated in the urine over the following 72 hours[32].

In women, the application of a single dose of 3 mg of 17β-oestradiol in a hydroalcoholic solvent leads to a plasma E_2 increase within

12 hours of administration. The plasma levels obtained vary considerably from one individual to another[33]. However, after three repeated daily applications, the mean plasma concentrations of E_2 become stable and reach levels of 110 ± 24 pg/ml, i.e. values within the follicular phase range[34] (Figure 15.2). No peak increments are observed, this being mainly due to the reservoir effect of the skin, which allows constant gradual diffusion of the steroid.

The E_2/E_1 ratio observed after percutaneous application of oestradiol gel remains around 1, close to the physiological values observed during the follicular phase of a normal cycle[13,19,25,34]. Levels of E_2 of around 100 pg/ml are able to relieve climacteric complaints and to prevent hypo-oestrogenic consequences[33,34]. The plasma levels of follicle-stimulating hormone (FSH) and luteinizing hormone (LH) exhibit a significant decrease[13,34], even if, as with other oestrogenic therapy, the gonadotrophins do not decrease to pre-menopausal levels. However, it is known that a decrease in plasma gonadotrophins is not necessary to obtain relief of climacteric complaints[35].

Efficacy of percutaneous oestradiol at the target level

The stable, proliferative-phase range plasma oestradiol values that are obtained correct oestrogen deficiency predictably and ensure efficacy of the treatment at the target level. The relief of hot flushes and night sweats is rapid, occurring within the first few days of treatment, and vaginal dryness is also reversed[33,34]. Psychological symptoms, particularly depressive mood, can be reversed provided the levels of plasma E_2 remain between 50 and 150 pg/ml[36].

As far as the endometrium is concerned, it was shown by Whitehead et al.[6] that percutaneous E_2 induced an increase in nuclear oestradiol receptors (REN) and soluble progesterone receptors (RPC) within the proliferative-phase range, demonstrating the efficacy of this therapy on the target organ. Thus, progestogen therapy should be added on a sequential basis to avoid endometrial hyperplasia, as with any other (active) oestrogenic therapy.

Finally, the activity of percutaneous oestradiol on the breast has not been assessed by *in vivo* studies. However, breast tenderness and mastodynia, which have been correlated with high oestradiol levels in pre-menopausal women[37], have been observed in some post-menopausal women treated with percutaneous oestradiol. In these

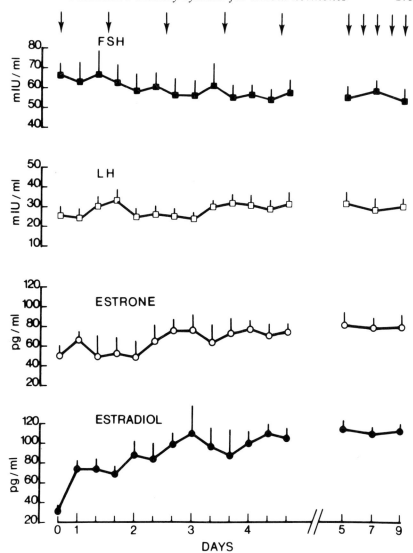

FIGURE 15.2 Basal serum concentrations (mean ± SEM) of follicle-stimulating hormone (FSH), luteinizing hormone (LH), oestrone (E_1) and oestradiol (E_2), and their incremental changes after daily percutaneous application of 5 g oestradiol gel in seven post-menopausal women (from Sitruk-Ware, R. et al.[34], with permission).

cases, E_2 plasma levels reached high values of over 150 pg/ml[38].

The percutaneous administration of oestradiol is also efficient in preventing osteoporosis. Recently, Riis et al.[39] clearly demonstrated by single and dual photon absorptiometry that bone mineral content remained constant in post-menopausal women treated for 2 years with percutaneous E_2, while calcium and placebo treated women had the same rate of loss of trabecular bone.

Hepatocellular effects of oestradiol: oral versus percutaneous administration

In a previous study conducted by our group percutaneous administration of oestradiol was not found to be associated with an increase in serum TG[40] as had been reported by other investigators in the case of vaginal rings[41] and implants[42]. This observation was related to the liver bypass. Other studies have been carried out which confirm the importance of the choice of route of administration of oestradiol to avoid metabolic effects.

Fåhraeus presented the results of his study in 38 post-menopausal women who received either oestradiol cream 5 g/day (i.e. 3 mg E_2) or oral micronized oestradiol (2 mg and subsequently 4 mg/day)[43,44]. He demonstrated that oral treatment raised HDL and decreased LDL levels – thus increasing the HDL/LDL ratio – and also elevated the TG concentration, whereas the percutaneous treatment did not induce any significant change in the lipoprotein pattern.

He indicated that the different effects of the two routes on lipoproteins might be explained by dissimilar plasma oestrogen profiles and differences in liver induction. He also showed that oral therapy preferentially increased the HDL2 fraction. He accordingly discussed a possible beneficial effect of oral therapy in that high HDL/LDL ratios reportedly offered protection against cardiovascular disease in the general population[45]. However, other potentially adverse effects of oral therapy might neutralize the supposedly 'beneficial' increase in the HDL/LDL ratio, these being an increase in TG, and alterations in plasma RS and clotting factors.

It was recently shown[25] that oral administration of 17β-oestradiol, the natural oestrogen, resulted in a substantial increase in E_1 levels and metabolic disturbances in the form of increases in sex-binding protein (SBP), RS and VLDL, and a decrease in AT III activity such as occurs with synthetic oestrogens (Figure 15.3). The same molecule administered parenterally did not induce these changes. Percutaneous administration of E_2 led to a physiological plasma E_2/E_1 ratio and did not induce any change in hepatic proteins.

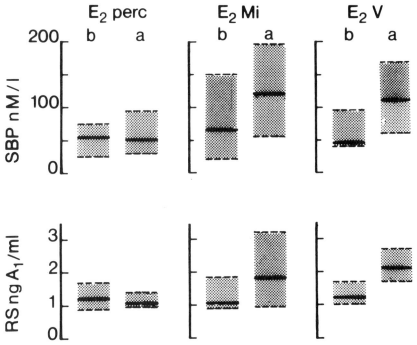

FIGURE 15.3 Median (and range) of plasma levels of sex-binding protein (SBP) and renin substrate (RS) before (b) and after (a) therapy in three groups of patients receiving either percutaneous oestradiol (E_2 perc) 3 mg/day, oral micro-ionized oestradiol (E_2 Mi) 2 mg/day, or oral oestradiol valerate (E_2 V) 2 mg/day (adapted from de Lignières, B. et al.[25])

Mode of administration and compliance to percutaneous therapy

For topical treatment 17β-oestradiol is dissolved in a hydroalcoholic solvent and presented in a gel form (60 mg of oestradiol per 100 g of gel). Each tube contains 80 g of gel. Calibration of the tube indicates quantities of 5 g of gel containing 3 mg of E_2. The gel is applied to the skin of the abdomen, arms or shoulders over a surface area in excess of 70 cm^2 and must be allowed to dry for five minutes after application. The patient is informed of the symptoms of both overdosing (mastodynia) and underdosing (persistence of night sweats). She is then able to modify the dose of oestrogens herself, although the finest control is achieved by plasma determinations. Women who have been informed about the side effects of oral therapy accept a new form of drug administration fairly well. Indeed, patients are usually less surprised by the mode of administration than the prescribing doctor, and the rate of compliance is very high, even on a long-term basis.

The transdermal therapeutic system

A new system for delivering E_2 through the skin was developed recently and is now on the market in Switzerland and the USA, and reaches the market in other countries.

The E_2 transdermal therapeutic system (TTS) consists of a thin multilayered unit containing a drug reservoir, a rate-controlling membrane and an adhesive layer[46]. TTS units have surface areas of 5, 10 or 20 cm^2 and they administer oestradiol at controlled rates of 0.025, 0.05 or 0.1 mg/day *in vivo*. Pharmacokinetic studies have shown that plasma E_2 rose from a pretreatment level of about 7 pg/ml to approximately 25, 40 or 75 pg/ml during the use of these systems, while E_1 rose to 30–60 pg/ml, ensuring an E_2/E_1 ratio of approximately 1, which is within the pre-menopausal range[46]. Steady-state levels can be obtained if the systems are worn for 72 hours and changed twice weekly[47]. A decrease in E_2 is immediately observed after removal of the system, suggesting loss of the 'reservoir effect'. The occlusive membrane greatly increases diffusion through the stratum corneum[30], thus achieving therapeutic efficacy with very low doses of E_2.

Utian presented the results of a large multicentre study carried out in the USA.

This randomized double-blind study involved 238 women with post-menopausal symptoms, who were treated with either Estraderm TTS or active Premarin plus a placebo TTS.

The efficacy of Estraderm was comparable with that of Premarin and hot flushes were relieved in most cases (Figure 15.4).

Endometrial biopsies were performed in women both before and after 18 weeks of therapy, at which stage 5 cases showed hyperplasia, indicating the rapid efficacy of the drug and the need to add sequential progestogen therapy. TTS tolerability was assessed by questionnaires sent out to the participating women, 70% of whom asked to remain on the medication.

Other clinical studies have shown that TTS-E_2 0.05 and 0.1 mg/day significantly reduced the frequency of hot flushes, had positive effects on vaginal cytology and did not induce any changes in the hepatic proteins, namely SBP, RS, thyroxine-binding protein (TBG) and corticosterone-binding globulin (CBG). Moreover, there were no significant changes in the urinary calcium/creatinine or hydroxyproline/creatinine ratios[48,49].

Endometrial studies have also shown proliferative effects after TTS-

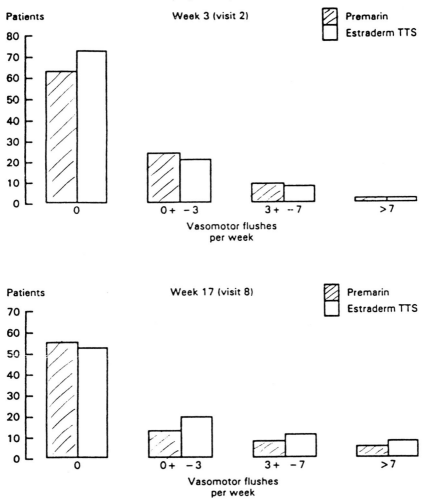

FIGURE 15.4 Number of hot flushes: comparison between pre-study control period (week 3) and last visit (week 17).
(From Nachtigall, L. and Utian, W. H. (1985). Proceedings of an International Symposium on Transdermal Estrogen. Berlin, West Germany)

E_2 0.05 mg/day used either alone or in combination with progestogens. No endometrial hyperplasia was observed[24].

Few skin reactions were reported; most were mild erythema and all were transient. They occurred with equal frequency in E_2 and placebo treatment groups[46].

The area of application of both percutaneous and transdermal systems should be changed regularly and not always be restricted to the same place. One reason for this is obvious in the case of TTS, since the occlusive membrane can lead to itching and transient skin irritation.

Another factor to be borne in mind is the potential effect of E_2 on adipose tissue growth. It has been shown that 17β-oestradiol stimulates the multiplication of human adipocyte precursors in culture[50]. However, in the long term clinical studies conducted to date no such effect has been reported *in vivo*.

Vaginal administration of steroids

The vaginal epithelium rapidly absorbs oestrone and oestradiol and the use of vaginal rings[41] or vaginal creams[51] leads to high plasma steroid values with physiological E_2/E_1 ratios.

Characteristics of Silastic devices: Devices made of dimethylpolysiloxane are nontoxic. They release the steroids they contain at a rate that is proportional to their surface area and inversely proportional to the thickness of their outer wall[52]. A vaginal ring developed by the Population Council for contraceptive purposes also appeared to be highly suitable for steroid administration through the vagina in the postmenopausal woman. In an effort to develop devices with more uniform release rates, the Population Council developed rings with a shell design. These shell rings have a steroid and Silastic layer applied around an inner core of inert Silastic. The active layer is covered with another layer of inert Silastic tubing, thus providing an almost uniform distance through which the steroid must travel in order to be absorbed[52,53].

Victor presented results obtained in women using vaginal rings delivering either E_2 alone or E_1 plus norgestrel. He showed that after some weeks of therapy the absorption of E_2 from the mucosa decreased even when new rings were inserted. Moreover, when E_2 was added to norgestrel, the absorption of the progestogen was decreased by the oestrogen. The explanation for this could be a rapid modification of the vaginal mucosa after therapy, leading to decreased permeability.

However, acceptability of the method was good even in cases of increased vaginal discharge. The advantage of the ring was mainly its long-lasting effect.

With these ring systems the mean oestradiol release rates were fairly constant ($152 \pm 21\ \mu$g per day with the 50 mm diameter ring and $183 \pm 34\ \mu$g per day with 58 mm systems).

The reservoir is sufficient to ensure effectiveness for at least six months[52].

This device has been demonstrated to be acceptable to women and to produce no significant metabolic effects, i.e. no changes in angiotensinogen, SBP or AT[41,52].

Implants

Subcutaneous implantation of oestradiol leads to a rise in plasma E_2 values and E_2/E_1 ratios close to physiological values. According to some authors the plasma levels increase to the proliferative-phase range and remain stable[42,54]. However, irregular absorption of the steroid may occur in some patients and once inserted the implants are difficult to remove in the event of overdosage or intolerance.

Studd proposed the implantation of subcutaneous devices delivering both oestradiol and testosterone. The advantages of this system are that it avoids the enterohepatic circulation and produces appropriate blood levels of E_2 and E_1 in a ratio of approximately 2 to 1. The technique was suitable for hysterectomy patients with an inadequate response to oral therapy or in cases where the woman complained of depression, loss of energy and loss of libido. However, it was stressed that testosterone is a potent androgen, able to stimulate clitoral and hair growth, which could induce very inconvenient side effects.

Conclusion

It is widely recognized that the oral administration of oestrogens is responsible for unfavourable metabolic side effects and many scientists have consequently focused their attention on parenteral routes of administration for oestradiol, mainly for use in women aged over 50. Percutaneous and transdermal therapies appear to be simple and safe methods of delivering oestrogens, since a natural molecule can be used, the plasma E_2 levels can be easily checked, and the therapy can be readily adjusted. The E_2/E_1 ratios obtained are physiological and no ultimate hepatic or metabolic toxicity has been observed. Such modes of administration represent a novel approach to the treatment of the climacteric woman and to all other forms of substitutive oestrogen therapy.

Alternative delivery systems which avoid the oral route can be proposed to the patient and her choice will be made on the basis of simplicity, acceptability, efficacy and freedom from toxicity.

The advances described and still further therapeutic improvements in alternative delivery systems for steroids will help to resolve the problems that can arise with menopausal replacement therapy and will yield positive benefits which will serve to improve both health and the quality of life throughout the post-menopausal years.

REFERENCES

1. Diczfalusy, E. (1984). Keynote address: Menopause and the developing world. In Notelovitz M., van Keep P. A. (eds.). *The Climacteric in Perspective*, p. 1–15. (Lancaster: MTP Press)
2. Weinstein, M. C. (1980). Estrogen use in post menopausal women. Cost, risks and benefits. *N. Engl. J. Med.*, **16**, 308
3. Utian, W. H. (1980). *Menopause in Modern Perspective*. (New York: Appleton Century Grafts)
4. Nachtigall, L. E., Nachtigall, R. H., Nachtigall, R. D. et al. (1979). Estrogen replacement therapy I: A 10-year prospective study in the relationship to osteoporosis. *Obst. Gynecol.*, **53**, 277
5. Gambrell, R. D. Jr. (1978). The prevention of endometrial cancer in postmenopausal women with progestogens. *Maturitas*, **1**, 107
6. Whitehead, M. I., Townsend, P. T., Pryse-Davies, J. et al. (1981). Effects of estrogens and progestins on the biochemistry and morphology of the postmenopausal endometrium. *N. Engl. J. Med.*, **305**, 1599
7. Stampfer, M. J., Williett, W. C., Colditz, G. A. et al. (1985). A prospective study of postmenopausal estrogen therapy and coronary heart disease. *N. Engl. J. Med.*, **313**, 1044
8. Bush, T. L. and Barrett-Connor, E. (1985). Non contraceptive estrogen use and cardiovascular disease. *Epidemiol. Rev.*, **7**, 80
9. Campbell, S. (1982). Potency and hepato-cellular effects of oestrogens after oral, percutaneous and subcutaneous administration. In van Keep P. A., Utian W. H. and Vermeulen A. (eds.). *The Controversial Climacteric*, pp. 103–125. (Lancaster: MTP Press)
10. Glueck, C. J., Fallat, R. W. and Scheel, D. (1985). Effects of estrogenic compounds on triglyceride kinetics. *Metabolism*, **24**, 537
11. Furman, R. H., Alaupovic, P. and Howard, R. P. (1967). Effect of androgens and estrogens on serum lipids and the composition and concentration of serum lipoproteins in normolipemic and hyperlipidemic states. *Progr. Biochem. Pharmacol.*, **2**, 215
12. Poller, L., Thompson, J. M. and Coope, J. (1977). Conjugated equine

estrogens and blood clotting: a follow-up report. *Br. Med. J.*, **1**, 935

13. Elkik, F., Gompel, A., Mercier-Bodard, C. et al. (1982). Effects of percutaneous estradiol and conjugated estrogens on the level of plasma proteins and triglycerides in post-menopausal women. *Am. J. Obst. Gynecol.*, **143**, 888

14. Mandel, F., Geola, F., Lu, J. et al. (1982). Biologic effects of various doses of ethinylestradiol in postmenopausal women. *Obstet. Gynecol.*, **59**, 673

15. Gordon, T., Kannel, W. B., Hjortland, M. C. et al. (1978). Menopause and coronary heart disease. The Framingham Study. *Ann. Intern. Med.*, **89**, 157

16. Stone, G. M., Baggett, B. and Donnelly, R. B. (1963). The uptake of tritiated estrogens by various organs of the ovariectomized mouse following intravenous administration. *J. Endocrinol.*, **27**, 271

17. Gallagher, T. F., Mueller, M. N. and Kappas, A. (1966). Studies on the structural basis for estrogen-induced impairment of liver function. *Medicine*, **45**, 471

18. Whitehead, M. I., McQueen, J., Minardi, J. et al. (1978). Clinical considerations in the management of the menopause: the endometrium. *Postgrad. Med. J.*, **54**, 59

19. Basdevant, A., de Lignières, B. and Guy-Grand, B. (1983). Differential lipemic and hormonal responses to oral and parenteral 17β-estradiol in post-menopausal women. *Am. J. Obstet. Gynecol.*, **147**, 77

20. Yen, S. S. C., Martin, P. L., Burnier, A. M. et al. (1975). Circulating estradiol, estrone and gonadotrophin levels following the administration of orally active 17β-estradiol in postmenopausal women. *J. Clin. Endocrinol. Metab.*, **40**, 518

21. Segot-Chicq, S., Teillaud, E. and Peppas, N. A. (1985). Les dispositifs à libération contrôlée pour la délivrance des principes actifs médicamenteux. I. Intérêt et applications. *STP PHARMA*, **1**, 25

22. Ryan, K. J. and Engell, L. L. (1953). The interconversion of estrone and estradiol by human tissue slices. *Endocrinology*, **52**, 287

23. Whitehead, M. I. (1982). Comparative studies of oral, vaginal, subcutaneous and percutaneous oestrogen administration on plasma oestrogen levels, SHBG and endometrial receptors. In van Keep P. A., Utian W. H. and Vermeulen A. (eds.). *The Controversial Climacteric*, pp. 110–116. (Lancaster: MTP Press)

24. Whitehead, M. I., Padwick, M. L., Endacott, J. et al. (1985). Endometrial responses to transdermal estradiol in postmenopausal women. *Am. J. Obstet. Gynecol.*, **152**, 1079

25. De Lignières, B., Basdevant, A., Thomas, G. et al. (1986). Biological effects of estradiol-17β in postmenopausal women: oral versus percutaneous administration. *J. Clin. Endocrinol. Metab.*, **62**, 536

26. Verheugen, C., Pardridge, W. M., Judd, H. L. et al. (1984). Differential permeability of uterine and liver vascular beds to estrogens and estrogen

conjugates. *J. Clin. Endocrinol. Metab.*, **59**, 1128

27. Steingold, K. A., Cefalu, W., Pardrige, W. et al. (1986). Enhanced hepatic extraction of estrogens used for replacement therapy. *J. Clin. Endocrinol. Metab.*, **62**, 761

28. Scheuplein, R. J. (1980). Percutaneous absorption: Theoretical aspects. In Mauvais-Jarvis P., Vickers C. F. H. and Wepierre J. (eds.). *Percutaneous Absorption of Steroids*, pp. 1–17. (London: Academic Press)

29. Mashchak, C. A., Lobo, R. A., Dozono-Takano, R. et al. (1982). Comparison of pharmacodynamic properties of various estrogen formulations. *Am. J. Obstet. Gynecol.*, **144**, 511

30. Vickers, C. F. H. (1980). Reservoir effect of human skin: pharmacological speculation. In Mauvais-Jarvis P., Vickers C. F. H. and Wepierre J. (eds.). *Percutaneous Absorption of Steroids*, pp. 19–29. (London: Academic Press)

31. Wendker, H., Schaefer, H. and Zesch, A. (1976). Penetration kinetics and distribution of topically applied estrogens. *Arch. Dermatol. Res.*, **256**, 67

32. Feldmann, R. J. and Maibach, H. I. (1969). Percutaneous penetration of steroids in man. *J. Invest. Dermatol.*, **52**, 89

33. Basdevant, A. and de Lignières, B. (1980). Treatment of menopause by topical administration of estradiol. In Mauvais-Jarvis P., Vickers C. F. H. and Wepierre J. (eds.). *Percutaneous Absorption of Steroids*, pp. 249–258. (London: Academic Press)

34. Sitruk-Ware, R., de Lignières, B., Basdevant, A. et al. (1980). Absorption of percutaneous oestradiol in postmenopausal women. *Maturitas*, **2**, 207

35. Utian, W. H., Katz, M., Davey, D. A. et al. (1978). Effect of premenopausal castration and incremental dosages of conjugated equine estrogens on plasma follicle-stimulating hormone, luteinizing hormone and estradiol. *Am. J. Obstet. Gynecol.*, **132**, 297

36. De Lignières, B. and Vincens, M. (1982). Differential effects of exogenous oestradiol and progesterone on mood in post-menopausal women: individual dose/effect relationship. *Maturitas*, **4**, 67

37. Sitruk-Ware, R., Sterkers, N. and Mauvais-Jarvis, P. (1979). Benign breast diseases. I. Hormonal investigation. *Obstet. Gynecol.*, **53**, 457

38. De Lignières, B. and Mauvais-Jarvis, P. (1981). Hormonal dependence of benign breast disease, gynecomastia and breast cancer. In Hollman K. H. , de Brux J. and Verley J. M. (eds.). *New Frontiers in Mammary Pathology*, pp. 287–308. (New York: Plenum Press)

39. Riis, B., Thomsen, K. and Christiansen, C. (1987). Does calcium supplementation prevent postmenopausal bone loss? A double-blind controlled clinical study. *N. Engl. J. Med.*, **316**, 173

40. Loeper, J., Loeper, J., Ohlgiesser, C. et al. (1977). Influence de l'estrogénothérapie sur les triglycérides. *Nouv. Press Méd.*, **6**, 2447

41. Mishell, D. R. Jr., Moore, D. E. and Roy, S. (1978). Clinical performance of endocrine profile with contraceptive vaginal rings containing a combination of estradiol and d-norgestrel. *Am. J. Obstet. Gynecol.*, **130**, 55

42. Greenblatt, R. B. and Brynner, J. R. (1977). Estradiol pellet implantation

in the management of menopause. *J. Reprod. Med.*, **18**, 307

43. Fåhraeus, L., Larsson-Cohn, U. and Wallentin, L. (1982). Lipoproteins during oral and cutaneous administration of oestradiol-17β to menopausal women. *Acta Endocrinol.*, **101**, 597

44. Fåhraeus, L. and Wallentin, L. (1983). High density lipoprotein subfractions during oral and cutaneous administration of 17β-estradiol to menopausal women. *J. Clin. Endocrinol. Metab.*, **56**, 797

45. Gordon, T., Castelli, W. P., Hjortland, M. C. et al. (1977). High density lipoprotein as a protective factor against coronary heart disease. *Am. J. Med.*, **62**, 707

46. Place, V. A., Powers, M., Darley, P. et al. (1985). A double-blind comparative study of Estraderm and Premarin in the amelioration of post menopausal symptoms. *Am. J. Obstet. Gynecol.*, **152**, 1092

47. Powers, M. S., Schenkel, L., Darley, P. E. et al. (1985). Pharmacokinetics and pharmacodynamics of transdermal dosage forms of 17β-estradiol: comparison with conventional oral estrogens used for hormone replacement. *Am. J. Obstet. Gynecol.*, **152**, 1099

48. Laufer, L., De Fazio, L., Lu, J. et al. (1983). Estrogen Replacement Therapy (ERT) by transdermal estradiol administration. *Am. J. Obstet. Gynecol.*, **146**, 533

49. Padwick, M. L., Endacott, J. and Whitehead, M. I. (1985). Efficacy, acceptability and metabolic effects of transdermal estradiol in the management of postmenopausal women. *Am. J. Obstet. Gynecol.*, **152**, 1085

50. Roncari, D. A. K. and Van, R. L. R. (1978). Promotion of human adipocyte precursor replication by 17β-estradiol in culture. *J. Clin. Invest.*, **60**, 503

51. Rigg, L. A., Hermann, H. and Yen, S. S. C. (1978). Absorption of estrogens from vaginal creams. *N. Engl. J. Med.*, **298**, 195

52. Roy, S. and Mishell, D. R. (1983). Current status of research and development of vaginal contraceptive rings as a fertility control method in the female. *Res. Front. in Fertil. Regul.*, **2**, 1

53. Victor, A. and Johansson, E. D. B. (1976). Plasma levels of d-norgestrel and ovarian function in women using intravaginal rings impregnated with d-norgestrel for several cycles. *Contraception*, **14**, 215

54. Thom, M. H., Collins, W. P. and Studd, J. W. W. (1981). Hormonal profiles in postmenopausal women with subcutaneous implants. *Br. J. Obstet. Gynecol.*, **88**, 426

Index

acetylation of POMC peptides, 4,5
adrenergic agonists, 110–12
adrenocorticotrophin (ACTH), 3–6,
   8–9
aging, changes caused by, 9–10
   see also menopause, biological
   changes at
alcohol, 9
Alzheimer's disease, 9
anabolic steroid therapy, 133–4
androgen
   levels in elderly males, 86–91
   therapy, 34, 42, 48
andropause, 85–91
animal models for inducing ovarian
   cancer, 33–5
antipsychotic activity, 4
anxiety, 10, 42, 48, 55, 61, 102, 137,
   156–8
artificial insemination by donor (AID),
   71
atherosclerosis, 60
   see also cardiovascular disease
avoidance behaviour, 4–8, 140, 143–4

behaviour
   abnormal, 9
   effect of peptides on, 4–9
blood pressure, effect of oestrogen
   therapy on, 97–9
bone density measurement techniques,
   128–30
bone loss, 46–7, 55, 66–8, 76, 115,
   125–34
   diagnostic techniques of ascertaining,
   128–30
   epidemiological studies of, 66–8, 76,
   126–8, 131–2
   prevention of, 46–7, 77, 97, 115,
   130–1, 132–4, 169

risk factors for, 126, 133
treatment of, 132–3
   see also osteoporosis
brain
   disturbances in functions of, 11
   effect of aging on, 9
breast cancer
   effect of hormones taken during
   pregnancy or for contraception,
   21–2, 27
   effect of menopausal hormones, 22–8
   risk of, 21–8, 61, 97, 104, 115
breast disease, benign, 26, 27
bromocriptine, 112–13

calcitonin, 3, 131, 132–4
calcitonin-gene-related peptide
   (CGRP), 3, 103
calcium, 3, 46, 55, 126–7, 131, 132–3,
   176
cancer
   endometrial, 26, 31–2, 44–6, 57–8,
   61, 97, 101, 116
   of breast, 21–8, 61, 97, 104, 115
   ovarian, 31–6
carbohydrate tolerance, 102, 103
cardiovascular disease, 47, 55–6, 59–60,
   67–71, 95–104, 170, 176
castration, 67, 69–71, 76–7
   see also oophorectomy
central nervous system effects of
   neuropeptides, 6–9
cholecystokinin-like peptides, 4
climacteric, 40–1
   in males, 85–91
   psychosocial research on, 155–67
   syndrome, 10, 42, 55, 61
clonidine, 110–12, 113
coagulation factors, 99
conception during peri-menopause, 40

187